As far as I know, her earlier experiments in technique as well as her later synthesis of them, have largely gone unrecorded. In her memory and for our sakes, we should see what we can piece together of how she went about training a dancer to become a therapeutic person.

Jarl E. Dyrud

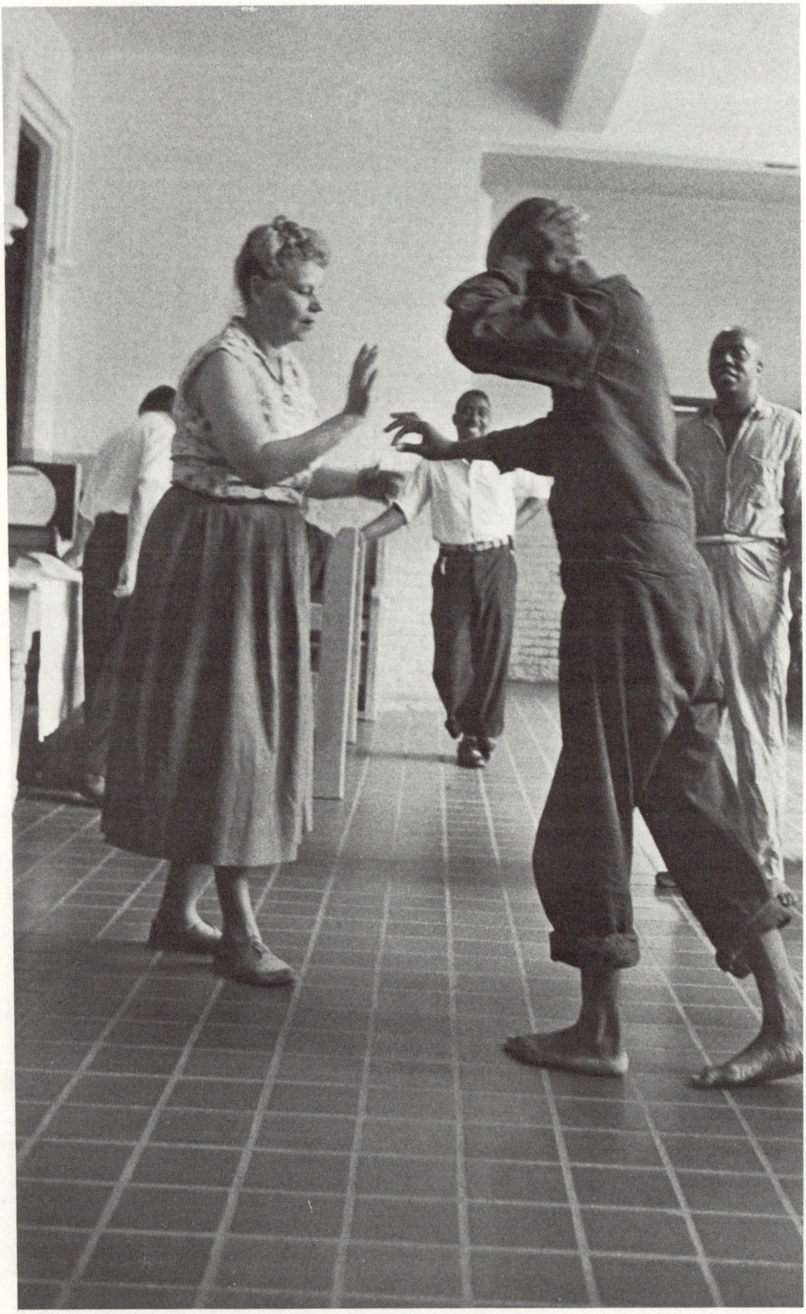

MARIAN CHACE:
HER PAPERS

Edited By
HARRIS CHAIKLIN

AMERICAN DANCE THERAPY ASSOCIATION

Library of Congress Catalog Number: 75-28984
ISSN 0065-8022
ISBN 0-915126-04-4

Acknowledgments

The editor wishes to thank the Marian Chace Memorial Fund which substantially made this book possible. In truth, all those who contributed are co-editors. The Marian Chace Memorial Fund is a non-profit, tax-deductible fund maintained by the American Dance Therapy Association. It is meant to be an ongoing tribute to Marian Chace by furthering education and scholarship in the field of dance therapy.

The editor gratefully acknowledges a generous contribution made in memory of James Hart Freudenthal which helped make publication of this volume possible.

TABLE OF CONTENTS

FOREWORD

Here are the papers of Marian Chace. They are in five sections: I, Biographical; II, Published; III; Panel Discussions; IV Unpublished; and V About. Within each section the material is presented in order of appearance. It was decided to keep introductory comment and explanation to a minimum. The papers speak for themselves.

It would be nice to say that this is a definitive edition; but it isn't. Anyone who knew Marian also knows that you had to work for what you learned from her. Collecting these papers was no exception. Marian never left a complete bibliography and she never used a footnote. Compiling this material was like trying to put a jigsaw puzzle together when you had no border pieces to frame the problem. My hope is that this initial collection will inspire others to complete the job.

Of course there are more people to thank than I can list here. I should like to mention Wynelle Delaney, Ann Lohn, Sister Christine Corey, and the Chestnut Lodge Library. They were helpful in locating written material and in checking bibliography. To the members of the ADTA who have waited so long and patiently for this I owe a special debt of gratitude. The book would have been completed sooner but twenty-three foundations and government granting agencies turned down requests for help. I believe Marian's papers will show them how wrong they were.

HARRIS CHAIKLIN

Columbia, Maryland
June 1975.

PART I

Biography; Auto, Professional, and Otherwise

The biography of Marian Chace remains to be written. She did leave partial statements, notes, and comments about the way her life had influenced her work. We have made selections from this material to illuminate Marian's professional development. They are not intended to present a coherent picture of her life; rather they are selected to reflect Marian's insight into the sources of her creative energy. In addition we present some notes from a journal Marian's mother kept.

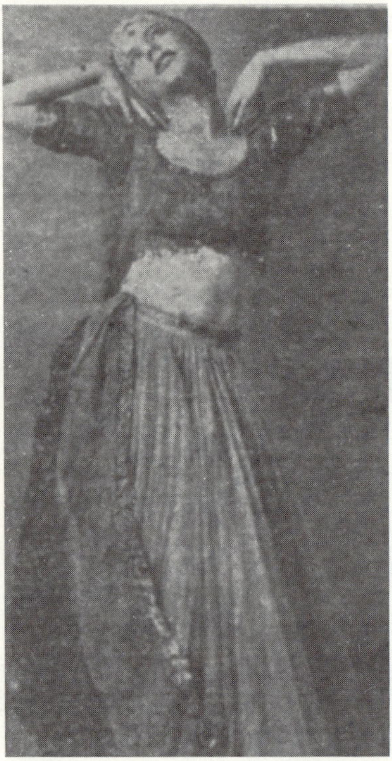

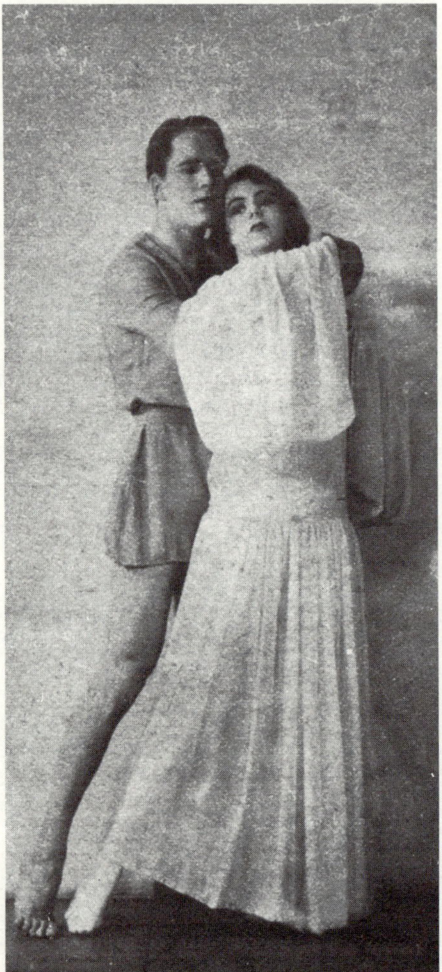

Mother's Journal

Marian Chace was born on October 31, 1896. About sixteen months later there was the following entry:

On Feb. 26 the long looked for event happened and Marian started bravely out to walk alone. For two months and more she had walked perfectly when somebody held one hand. For two or three weeks she had walked alone if someone walked directly back of her with hands held out each side where she could see them. Five or six feet, from one person to another, was all she could be induced to attempt entirely by herself. But on this eventful day up at Grandma Northrop's after walking between grandma and mamma who were on opposite sides of the room, baby suddenly started to go around the table which was in the centre of the room. This she did several times stopping now and then at mamma or grandma for a fresh start. Then off she walked into an adjoining room stopping at the nearest chair. When we went home she repeated her efforts. She was applauded roundly. I shall never forget the half-delighted, half afraid little laugh by which she showed her appreciation of her new attainment. In four days she learned to walk freely all over the house alone, stand alone, get up from a sitting or fallen position on the floor without touching any object for support, stoop down pick up an object from the floor and regain the erect position without change of base, and walk easily while carrying something in her arms which prevented them from being used as aids in balance. Some of these things many babies do before walking but Marian never attempted any of them until she could walk alone.

Affection [from the same time]

There has been a marked increase in demonstration of affection during the past three weeks. Voluntary loving in her baby way—laying her head down on the face or hand or knee of the one loved and saying "ah"—is very frequent. Kisses are given only on request.

Motion

Marian is fond of rhythmical motion, loving to be danced with to the sound of music. She also takes hold of her dress and shakes it up and down when she hears music while standing, or jumps up and down shaking her arms if sitting.

APRIL 1898

April 1

Is fond of imitating facial expressions. She grins and scowls in imitation of aunt Mable. Imitated pat-a-cake and an original little finger play of her mother's.

April 2

Last week I gave Marian a little elastic band. She played with it stretching it out and letting it relax and I told her the name, elastic. A moment or two afterwards I noticed her pull up her dress and lay the band on the top of her stocking. This she did a number of times while I wondered what was the reason. Finally I remembered that I have called her hose supporters elastics. She associated the two.

[*DEVELOPMENTAL HISTORY*]

Nov. 20 Syllabus No. 1 1898

Barnard

Name Marian Chace
Date of Birth Oct. 31, 1896

Physical Characteristics

1. Slight, medium strength, good color but not rosy
2. *Gait* Firm and graceful
3. *Health* Excellent
4. *Bodily Defects* Ears not exactly alike. One nearly resembling her mother's and one her father's.

Characteristics of Environment

1. *Parents*
   Nationality—American
   Occupation—Newspaper reporter
   Disposition—Excitable, sensitive, hopeful—versus sad, sympathetic, *reticent*.
2. *Home*
   Location—City—good street
   Health conditions—seem all right
   Possessions
      Pets—Cat in the house
      Toys—Dolls, blocks, dishes, tin kitchen, doll carriage, doll's bed

Books—Picture books

Companions—Few cousins, older. Plays best with ones seven and nine years old.

Playground

Summer time—Down the river, lawn or cottage piazza.

Winter—house

Experiences

Journeys—To Inonocontang
To Block Island

Illnesses—Convulsions twice,—arm out of joint,—stomach trouble two days once.

Changed residence—Down river and back.

3. *Characteristics of temperament and disposition*

Excitable, energetic but not very noisy, confiding, sensitive, happy, sympathetic, stubborn, slightly selfish but yields to persuasion, honest, courageous, leader at home with younger children, follower of older children.

Affections

Strong for papa, momma and relatives, for animals, sea (doubt if it is the sea itself or the pleasure derived from throwing stones in the waves) and especially for her dolls. Likes books.

Characteristics of mind

1. Perception
   Color
   Sound
   Form
   Motion
   Number
   Which sense is best?
2. Memory
   Of incidents in child's own life—Ordinary happenings she does not talk about much herself but is almost always able to answer questions and often supplements the recital with her own version. A visit to the menagerie at Roger Williams Park she talked about for a couple of weeks with great enthusiasm. When Block Island is mentioned she talks about the boat, the beach, throwing stones in the water etc.
   Of ideas—
   Of dreams—
   Of punishment—Effective

Of injustice or ill treatment
Of pleasant experiences—Good
Rote memory—Untried

Imagination

Very strong
Mostly concerning her doll or going down street, or going to the store. Imagines the possession and distribution of candy or some favorite article of diet.
One night she was playing "go down street" and went gleefully into an adjoining room. In a moment she returned with a very sad face and in a most disconsolate tone said "Missed the car." She had been out with her grandma and mother more than a week before when they missed the car. Nothing had been said about the matter since. Hanging her hat up on a chair she said "Wait 'nother car." This was entirely original.

Expression

In play. Symbolic—No pleasure in block building unless something particular is being made, as a house, dog's house, steps, cars, etc.
In manual work—Very careful, blocks must be straight, coverings on dolls bed straight etc.

Language

Vocabulary—large, readily enlarged.

Responsiveness

Love—decidedly
Will—how shown?

Autobiographical Fragments

Marian made several starts at a biographical statement. She never got very far. Each one she did added something new. While there is some repetition in the statements included here, their differing contexts add some understanding of the creative genie Marian struggled with.

1

My dance career started by doing small concerts in Washington and then in places such as towns in Virginia and North Carolina.

I was studying rhythmic dance with a group who occasionally performed at civic events.

I felt the need of more formal work and went to the New York School of Denishawn for the summer. I intended to return to Washington, but instead I married and went on a vaudeville tour across country. My husband was a Denishawn dancer and we had our own "act". My teachers at that time included Martha Graham and Paul Mathis. Before leaving for our tour we were married at the "Little Church Around the Corner" and had a wedding reception at the school.

When we reached California we stayed until after our daughter was born. We then returned to the East. We stayed in Washington for awhile dancing and teaching.

Ted Shawn, Miss Ruth and the Denishawn Company was touring through parts of Asia. They returned a year later and toured with a company of the Ziegfeld Follies. My husband and I joined them and went to the summer school.

The following fall we continued at Denishawn House as members of the Company and lived at Denishawn House. Our daughter lived with my parents in Washington at this period.

After four years, Mr. Shawn and Ruth St. Denis went their separate ways and at Mr. Shawn's plan with us we went back to Washington to open a school and develop our dance group.

Then followed many years of teaching, doing choreography for the group performing and all the things connected with these activities.

The group which performed was first of all well trained dance wise and then directed as performers. The school as a whole was not involved. It was a tremendous satisfaction to do the choreography for the group to perform.

During the first years my first interest was my own dancing. However, as time moved on I became more interested in group interaction than in solo performance. The dances were concerned with problems of people. I was interested in movement portraits for my own solo performances. My last major group ballet was called American Horizons and contained a satire on the five—four decisions of the Supreme Court. The dancers wore legal robes and wigs and masks of stylized portraits of members of the Supreme Court.

I was in the process of dancing roles of women of history when I gave up the group and closed the school.

When I was first in Washington, I was interested only in the people capable of creative work and training. However, concomitant with my interest in group interaction in composition I grew interested in the action and interaction of people who were awkward, lacking in ability to move with rhythm and with efficient coordination. I became interested in what they found in group dance action to help them to feel at ease.

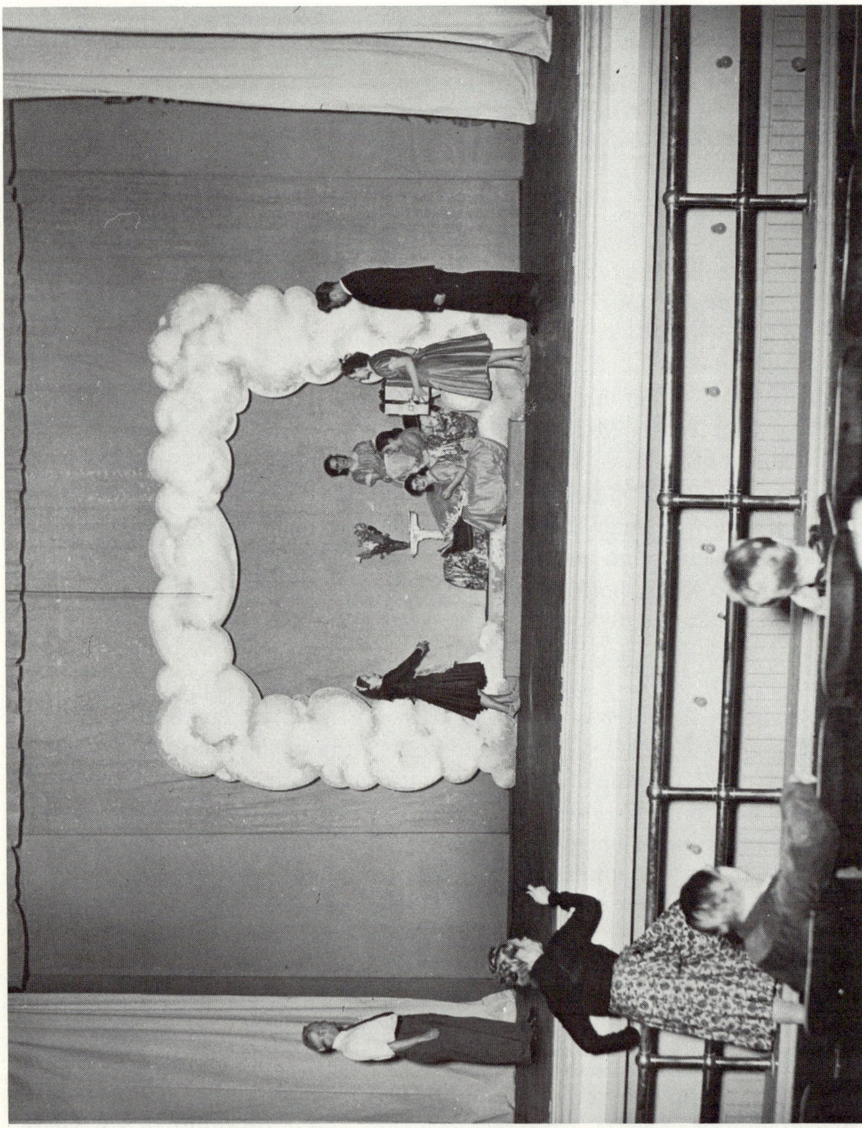

2

Dance therapy, as a discipline, did not move into the mental hospital full blown and as a bright idea to be sold. Its roots were in work that had been going on for many years prior to this in the community. As with all new approaches to problems of human beings, there is a tendency toward a way of thinking, out of the needs of the individual.

My own reasons for starting to dance made one aware of dance as a tool other than for performing. My back had been injured in a dive. The tension in the back muscles when I painted, which was my means of creative expression, caused my hand to lack sureness, which was discouraging. At the suggestion of my doctor, I used dance for a creative outlet and as an aid for relaxing and strengthening my back muscles. I had always danced, but I had thought of painting as a career. However, I soon found that dance was my natural means of communication in creative forms.

One paragraph must cover my development as a dancer although this is the development that enabled me to use dance as a tool for communication with people who were blocked in verbal expression. I was soon performing in concerts as both an individual and as a group member on a professional level. Then came the years at Denishawn where I was under the influence of Ted Shawn and Ruth St. Denis as mentors and teachers. As a member of the company and as a teacher in the school, my former husband, Lester Shafer, and I lived at Denishawn House and I was enriched through them and their many friends in the fields of the arts. There I learned that there is not one way of moving, but an infinite number of ways depending upon one's cultural background as well as religious and philosophical motivation. I learned to function as a group member, with ideas of others and as a soloist with my own ideas or those of my former husband.

The broad and eclectic approach of the school at Denishawn at that time enabled the pupils to find their own way of moving and developed their own abilities as choreographers and teachers as well as performing dancers. One was never taught a particular way of moving without having it related to the folk culture from which it came. The combination of modified ballet forms, contemporary dance, Dalcroze and other technical forms developed body equipment to use flexibly for whatever ideas were to be developed.

I had never considered anything other than to be a performing dancer. However, my former husband and I felt it important to return to Washington where our small daughter was living with my family. Since Ted Shawn wished to have a branch of Denishawn in Washington, we were able to combine our performing and teaching in a school still centered on the concepts in which we both believed.

Many people, even those who speak glibly about dance therapy, are unaware of the beginnings and the reasons for the direction of the use of rhythmic action as a tool for communication with mental patients. They are also unaware that this use as a therapeutic tool was not a bright idea to be sold to the staff and patients in the hospital. My use of movement for communication and meeting needs was already recognized in Washington before I tried reaching people in a hospital setting.

There were many people who came to my dance studio who were neither potentially artist dancers, nor people well equipped in fine coordination of muscular development. Some came on their own, some were sent by doctors or clinics. There were both adults and children. Yet all of these people had a great need to dance with others and to learn more about their own body movements.

3

As a concert dancer and choreographer I had, of course, had an interest and training in the dynamics of the use of movement for communication of ideas and feeling as an art form. At the moment that I became interested in the reasons for seeking dance as an outlet by the non-dancers coming to the school, I added another dimension to my interest and teaching. I began to use my training as a means of communication and body awareness rather than as a teacher of art forms. As the pupils in this group made application and then participated in the first class, I observed and empathized with the needs being expressed.

Loneliness was always expressed. After this, many other emotions were stated. Too frequently, people expressed a feeling of inadequacy, an unworthiness and a feeling of awkwardness in their bodies which made it difficult to relate to others. Others who seemed quite shy in talking, would express such extreme aggressiveness in action that they would, of course, be shunned. But all were seeking something nameless to them which would help them to relate. In speech this is always difficult to observe as speech so frequently disguises what is really being said.

Studying and empathizing with people's expression of needs was for the purpose of trying to supply those things for which they were asking. This thrust has continued throughout the development of the use of body action for communication with mental patients.

Through this support for people asking help for human needs rather than wishing to or having the expectation of becoming a creative dancer, the school gradually became divided into two groups of pupils. There were those receiving support and development as dancers and those receiving support in gaining more confidence and awareness of themselves as human beings. All of this began to take place in the early thirties.

There was direct reflection of my new awareness in my teaching and direction of the concert group. There seemed to be a greater freedom for creativity in the concert group, more alertness in the student body as a whole, both adults and children and a growing confidence in the people with difficulties who had come asking for help. There seemed to be real growth in the pupils throughout the school. I didn't realize that techniques for reaching schizophrenic patients were developing.

From the middle thirties until I moved for full time work in the hospital setting, pupils were sent to me by pediatricians, clinics and other physicians. I have this experience. I believe the techniques which were later called dance therapy came from directly thinking about the supplying of help for the needs of these people rather than merely absorbing them into classes with the usual goals in such classes.

In the children's group, there were problems of great shyness which prevented the children from relating to their peer group as well as children with problems of rebellion against authority to point of dismissal from their schools. There were others with severe difficulty in muscle action. In the adult group there were some pupils who were post-hospital patients who interested me a great deal.

By 1940, the student body was almost equally divided between those being trained in dance as such and those needing help as people. It was in the late thirties. I was asked to open a dance clinic by the D.C. Medical Society. This I refused to do for many reasons.

It is interesting that training of various groups developed concomitantly with my own gaining of further knowledge and more sureness in working with the student body. I spoke frequently to various parent-teacher groups at their request on the value of continuing the participation of children in dance as an important aspect of living in their development and growth. There were a number of classes held under the auspices of parent-teacher groups.

The next development in training was a request from a group of District of Columbia elementary school teachers for a ten week seminar in the use of rhythmic action for children who have specific problems. I used children who had come to my school for these various problems to demonstrate. The children found this very exciting and satisfying. I have followed this technique down through the years. I have found that those who have been helped are the ones who know what happened. After the end of the first year of these sessions, I was asked to continue on following years. Unfortunately, my involvement in the mental hospital setting, forced me to stop these sessions after three years.

Although many individuals were sent to me and I had been working in a school for children whose families were divorced and rejecting these children, I was not sure that the dance as non verbal communication was generally useful. All pupils with whom I had had contact had been predisposed to an interest. They either came on their own or had been sent by doctors, teachers, or parents, by people who were concerned directly with them. Therefore, for purposes of my own seeking, I made an opportunity to hold sessions with the adolescents in the National Training School for Girls, where the young people were sent after they had had serious trouble with the law. I found the same response that I had found with people for whom the sessions had been prescribed.

My next venture was holding classes for children and adolescents in one of the orphanages in Washington. All of this was a period of intense learning and observation and evaluating what happened during sessions of rhythmic action for building self respect, and non verbal communication. I wanted and found many varied contacts with people with as many varied problems and difficulties.

My days were divided and very full with both the clinical and the more usual dance sessions. Concomitantly, the dance group had developed tremendously and I was equally absorbed in training the dancers and composing choreography for the group. Here too, I had developed in the ability to help them to communicate in a valid way with their performing. We were constantly involved in many hours of rehearsals and performances.

In June of 1942 I started at Saint Elizabeths Hospital with a dance program. We still did not call it dance therapy. We spoke of it only as dance for communication.

I had worked with the daughter of a well known writer about psychiatry. She knew Dr. Overholser, who knew of my work. He asked if I would try the dance action with the patients. At my first interview, it was pointed out that I would not be able to work in a group, but they were interested in the work in body coordination which they had heard about.

This was before the days of group work with psychotic patients. I almost left, feeling that I did not belong there. I believed so strongly in group interaction that I would return to my studio where this was developing. However, since a few selected patients were involved in psychodrama sessions in the psychodrama theater, I was permitted to start sessions with this group. After two or three sessions, I was asked to give at least half my time on a salary instead of as a volunteer.

I was still not ready to give up the studio and my performing group. I felt that I must know about responses of patients in a ward setting.

Although at that time it was not usual to permit a volunteer to try a completely new type of program on a ward with patients, it was thought immediately these sessions were useful. Other wards were added some men's wards and some women's. Dr. Overholser gave the program his full support. He was noted for supporting things that proved useful for the patients, even when not previously tested.

Then came evaluation of what was happening with the patients. Among the psychiatrists was Dr. Samuel Hamilton. I will never forget that day. His eyes were very piercing and keen, even though there was a warmth about him. He decided that this was a form of therapy which enabled a patient to communicate and be more aware of himself. It was effective with many patients.

It took me a year to be sure that there was not over-enthusiasm. That first year was a very satisfying one. Although I was at the hospital only a few hours a week, it was long enough to begin to be aware of the ways in which patients communicated in movement and become at home with them. I began to understand their verbal speech which was so often symbolic. Because of the enthusiasm of the doctors and other staff members, I was able to learn a great deal from them.

Frances Herriott, the psychodramatist under whom I worked, was very helpful with the sessions in the theater.

Altogether, it seemed right to give half time to the program. I started on salary with the Red Cross in June of the next year.

The program of dance, which I preferred having it called at that time, had become so widely accepted at that time the schedule was almost too crowded. There were many servicemen being cared for at the hospital at that time, and one could never do all that needed to be done.

In addition to conducting sessions with patients, training and teaching was one of my functions. Red Cross recreation workers were being trained for overseas posts, and I was involved in that program both as a lecturer and as a supervisor of their practical experience. Again I was called upon to teach my own concepts in the approach to patients.

It was during this year and the following one that I had my first personal contact with psychodrama. It was felt that I understood and could interpret the feelings of patients and their consequent behavior patterns. I played the roles of patients, those who were withdrawn, those who were hostile or those who were manic or depressed. These training sessions were held for both social workers and recreation workers. Many of these trainees came from the field of education or other professional fields but were not trained in the things that they were called upon to do.

Many servicemen were very fearful of relating and programs were developed for teaching ballroom steps, using group rhythms. Only gradually were they introduced to couple dancing, and then with student nurses or Red Cross workers as partners.

It was during this year that I recognized that one could not work on a half time basis. That it was necessary to be wholely involved, if anything were to be really achieved. I knew that I must give myself completely to working with mental patients in the hospital setting or return to my studio.

I was still performing and directing my concert group, composing and directing dances for the Catholic University spring musical and teaching a few classes. When I was at the hospital, I felt needed at the studio, and when I was at the studio I felt a need to be at the hospital.

When I was at the hospital, full time, many new programs were established and developed. A policy was established during this year that has always been adhered to. No program is established prior to consultation with the doctor in charge of the group of patients involved. Programs always fit into a doctor's goals. It has always been my point of view that this can be done without feeling one's own integrity damaged.

During this first year of full time work at Saint Elizabeths, many exciting events took place. Some of them were establishment of new programs with patients, some had to do with my own training and with some opportunities for feeling more involved with the hospital staff.

The doctor in charge of a group of men receiving electroshock therapy was willing to try a program of music and dance rhythms in conjunction with the shock treatment. Prior to the treatment, folk music, conversation and singing kept the men occupied. When they were resting following the treatment, a program of usually soft music was played. I learned what would keep them asleep, what could reduce restlessness if some were restless and what would wake them up for breakfast. Following a shower, the men would join in a group session of rhythmic action.

Another very exciting session was one with overactive and hostile patients, most of whom were unpredictable in mood and some were apt to be assaultive. The purpose of this session in addition to communicating was to reduce the activity. Here is where we would end the session in listening quietly to Bach music, a long distance from the screaming fidgiting and restless movement over the benches and pacing with anger.

A satisfying session was that held with very depressed and actively suicidal patients.

For myself, I learned how to communicate with and receive communications from patients with many different behavior patterns.

A session held after regular hours was with servicemen who had just arrived from the war front, both the Pacific and the Atlantic theaters. These men were confused, lost and filled with guilt. Here, one of the leading composer-pianists assisted in the program. We alternated between rhythmic movement, singing and often encouraging individuals to play, however inadequately, for themselves.

During this period, a great many psychiatrists who were training at that time and have since received much recognition were on the grounds. My understanding was greatly augmented. It was indeed a privilege to exchange ideas, concepts and theories with them. After watching a session, they would ask me questions. I would do the same thing and then we would have a discussion.

I began attending clinical conferences. These were held daily and one could learn a great deal, both from the discussion and the presentation of the patient. In addition, I took classes at the Washington School of Psychiatry. My courses were Basic Psychiatry, Adjunctive Therapies, Art

Therapy, and Assets of the Mentally Ill under Dr. Frieda-Fromm-Reichmann. These courses extended over a period of three years.

I began lecturing and doing demonstrations outside of Saint Elizabeths in 1956. During that year I spoke about dance therapy at Chestnut Lodge. The Therapists who were present questioned me at great length about my theories and techniques. After this session followed by a session with a group of patients, I was asked to give as much time as possible to Chestnut Lodge. I have been there continuously ever since.

I found that the work at both places was most helpful. Discussion with the therapists, relating to patients on a more individual basis has always been valuable in my own development, and enriched the program at Saint Elizabeths Hospital. From Saint Elizabeths, I took the work in groups. The two programs were mutually enriching.

My reading during the 40's and even to the present has had to be in other areas than dance. There has been a little written on the non verbal and a great deal that has been helpful in group dynamics. However, there has been almost nothing that one can add to one's knowledge in the area of body action in relation to communication.

4

The following article describes the early development of Marian Chace's professional involvement in dance therapy. It will be continued in a forthcoming issue. It is as yet untitled.

Untitled Article on Professional History

The basic principle of the discipline called dance therapy is an aware communication in non-verbal terms. Rhythmic action is the tool used by the therapist.

In attempting to give a history of its beginnings and development, I must go back to my school of dance in Washington, D. C.

After a number of years at Denishawn House in New York, as a member of the Company and teacher. I returned to Washington, my home, as co-director of a branch of Denishawn in 1930.

One problem in any dance school is the many pupils who are non-dancers. They have neither the physical equipment, the desire nor the drive to become dancers, and a teacher is often frustrated by attempting to absorb them into a class. My interest in people's need for communication in movement came from this frustration. What is it that people are seeking in movement with others and why, I continually asked myself, do these non-dancers continue to study, year after year, in the face of technical failure and the inability to perform publicly?

I began to be aware of the needs these people were expressing through their bodies. As I became increasingly involved in my interest, I spent many hours in contemplation, and I found the understanding of their communications more and more clear.

Out of observing the non-verbal communication of individuals taking their first classes, I begin to understand and meet the needs for which they were asking help. Instead of feeling frustrated when they lagged behind the more adequate pupils, I tried to empathize with them as people.

Obviously, my teaching was undergoing change. Unconsciously, my centering, for all pupils, became a support of them as people as well as dancers. While the students at the school found satisfaction in various ways, I think of the whole period of the 1930's for me as one of intense absorption in learning about non-verbal communication.

I was led in many directions through this absorption. I worked with people who came to the school on their own, with children from clinics, with children and adolescents in orphanages and special schools, with the young girls in the National Training School (a correctional institution), and with individuals sent by pediatricians, general practitioners, psychologists and psychiatrists.

At no time during this period, however, did I think in terms of a discipline which would be called "dance therapy." When, in the late thirties, Dr. Truman Abbe, a general practitioner and diagnostician in Washington, brought me a request from the District of Columbia Medical Society to open a clinic, I refused. I believed strongly in dance as an art form for communication (and I still do), but at that time I felt that a clinic would be an exploitation of dance, rather than another use of dance. It seems strange, in retrospect, that I once held such a view.

One aspect of the work at this period was important to the development and broadening of my concepts. Dr. Agnes Bruce Greig had founded a clinic for disturbed children. This has continued in Washington since her death and has now become the Agnes Bruce Greig School for children with emotional problems affecting their learning.

Dr. Greig became interested in the help children seemed to derive from participation in my dance classes. She observed that my pupils seemed to develop more confidence, became able to function with their peers in a more satisfactory way, and improved in their coordination. She recommended that some of her clinic children come to my studio as an adjunctive tool for her work.

Many of the children were fearful of participating in activity with their peers. Others were so hostile to authority that they were very difficult to control. One of her students was a mirror reader. As her body image improved and her self-respect developed, she was able to function properly and her reading generally, improved markedly.

Discussion of the problems and goals with Dr. Greig was invaluable to me in coming to understand how body action is related to emotional problems.

Among others, Dr. Cousins, a pediatrician, sent me many of his patients. Again, he would always discuss with me what he hoped would happen for these children. And, again, it was of untold value to me, not only in working with the children, but in checking my impressions of what they were communicating, non-verbally, in their classes with me.

In the late thirties, I worked with the first person who was a schizophrenic. She was not only a post hospital case, but she had arrested tuberculosis with concomitant physical problems that had to be taken into consideration, as well as her emotional difficulties. I was completely naive, and I was grateful for the medical guidance of her physician. His goal was that she develop more initiative so that she could function independently. This, of course, involved more awareness of self, more confidence and better coordination. Both she and her physician felt that our goal was accomplished through body-action communication and the consequent forming of satisfactory relationships.

I was asked to try dance action in the Silver Spring School, a special school for children rejected by their families because of the parents' divorce and remarriage. These children were lacking incentive in their classes, quarrelsome and rebels against authority.

As I worked with them, there seemed to be a strong correlation between improved body action and physical coordination, and their concentration and learning ability in academic class work. The teachers felt that the situation was also helped through the youngsters' finding a group feeling with one another in movement. There was such a marked change in the class work, that it was decided to evaluate this through continuing objective tests. Unfortunately, the findings were only discussed and not written.

Out of this experience, I was eager to learn if some of the adolescents in the National Training School for girls would respond to dance action as an adjunct to rehabilitation. In spite of the fact that it was a punitive environment at that time, respect for themselves seemed to develop among these young women through improved body action.

I worked with them for only a few months. Even the social workers felt that little could be done for them on a permanent basis while the punitive atmosphere, rather than a concentration on rehabilitation, remained. I left, not because of discouragement with the individuals, but I was upset at the environment, about which I could do nothing. But, again, I had observed the value of rhythmic action as a tool for self-respect and communication, even in a defeating environment.

Immediately following the experience in the National Training School, I began to hold classes in an orphanage in Washington. I saw these classes as an added learning experience with people who had problems different from any I had yet worked with.

Among these children and adolescents was an underlying feeling of being outside of the community. The counselors and teachers were warm and well-trained people who were working on the children's development and growth in an institutional setting. The same benefits already observed from improved coordination, self-respect and the feeling of groupness proved useful here, too.

During this whole period, I spent many hours in contemplation, in attempts to understand what happened to people when they moved together in a creative way. Many concepts I developed came into use later in working with schizophrenic and other psychotic patients.

I became convinced that there are two levels of communication between people; the non-verbal and the verbal. Moreover, I learned that the non-verbal is a direct form of communication which cannot be disguised. Verbal speech can be used to augment the non-verbal, as a disguise of true feelings, or it may have no relationship to true feeling.

I learned that the non-verbal communication is always present, and that it is not enough for the leader to understand what is being said by another. The leader must be sufficiently alert and aware of the responses of his own musculatures to know what he is communicating and how his non-verbal communication is affecting others in the group. I learned that interaction in a group is often more useful than in a one-to-one relationship.

Perhaps the thing that brought my learning experiences into focus most clearly was the obligation to speak to countless community groups about the need for continuing dance opportunity for children as they are growing and developing. These speaking engagements required that I formulate my ideas sufficiently clearly to articulate them to a general audience.

Then, each year for three years before I began using dance action in the hospital setting, I held a ten-week, once-a-week seminar for school teachers, at their request, in the use of body action with children who had special problems. For these sessions it was necessary to be so sure of what I believed and so clear in expressing it, that I could communicate it in a teaching role to the professional educators.

I do not wish to imply that my school was entirely clinical. By the time I gave full time to my work in the hospital, it was perhaps fifty percent clinical. But through the years, I was interested in dance as an art form and a theater medium. Denishawn classes, rehearsals with the performing group, dance concerts under civic sponsorship and the University of Virginia, dance direction for the Catholic University of America's spring musicals and many other activities using dance as an art form absorbed at least half of my time.

My interest in the presentation of ideas through dance, with a performing group of concert caliber developed through a dozen years of hard work, was a difficult thing to give up. However, my growing awareness and understanding of the therapeutic value of dance as nonverbal communication was a compelling influence.

About 1940, I began to teach the daughter of Edith Stern, a writer in the psychiatric field. She was a friend of Dr. Winfred Overholser, Superintendent of Saint Elizabeth's Hospital, a Federal psychiatric hospital in Washington, D. C. When she talked to him of my work with her daughter and others, he invited me to try it at the hospital.

Dr. Overholser was noted for giving a welcome to new ideas that showed promise. He had me contact Miss Margaret Hagen, field director of the Red Cross at the hospital. I started as a Red Cross volunteer in the psychodrama department directly under Miss Frances Herriott, psychodramatist, and indirectly under Dr. Roscoe Hall, chief of psychotherapy.

Dr. Hall, like Dr. Overholser, was very much interested in music, painting and all of the arts as a means of communication for patients, and all three of these people gave tremendous support to me as I began to work with a tool and technique never before attempted with the mentally ill in a hospital setting.

Professional Notes

Three brief selections are presented from the numerous notes Marian left. She was apparently in the habit of writing down her thoughts. The first were found in a little pad which contained a record of payments for dance classes at $2.00 a lesson, instructions for folk dances, notes from case conferences and other odds and ends. They were probably done in the late forties. And they represent a clear statement of Marian's belief that movement emanates from the center of the body.

The second set comes from about the same time. It should be read not as a finished product but rather as a rare glimpse of the process Marian went through as she developed her method. She never abandoned the issues identified here; the urgency to do something now, the knowledge that dance therapy would require a scientifically acceptable underpinning, and the ambivalence about seeing dance as a therapy.

The final piece is probably from an early presentation that Marian made.

1. MOVEMENT

All movement of the body is energy directed thru a given set of muscles away from a point of resistance. That visually satisfying movement called grace is merely efficiently directed muscular force. Awkwardness of movement that is unpleasant visually is misdirected muscular force. It does not matter whether one is speaking in terms of physical sports, dancing, or merely the acts in everyday life of walking, running, and sitting, the same principle holds true. It is in all cases the awkward mover who tires easily because of the waste energy he is expending to no purpose. In addition the person who moves ineffectually rarely uses a point of resistance to the given movement and so achieves practically no force or drive through his muscles regardless of the amount of energy expended. On the contrary the efficient mover expends a small amount of energy along a well defined track offers an equal resistance with the proper portion of his body and achieves the desired results with the minimum of a tiring effect.

Good posture is a result of efficient movement of the body or portions of the body through space. It is not something that can be developed by itself irrespective of the movement of the muscles of that body. The person who has round shoulders, lordosis, knock-knees, pigeon toes, a forward thrust head, or any of the numerous attributes of poor posture is merely an example of poor posture and extreme inefficiency of movement. As his muscles learn to function in action correctly, good posture will inevitably develop.

Rhythm in movement is proper timing of movement and not the result of some special aesthetic sense of the person moving. Rhythm is also a by-product of the ability to move efficiently and is not a special way of moving. Naturally no action, no matter how simple, is completely efficient when not properly timed. Conversely no timing of a movement, however complex, in relation to a specific sport such as tennis, golf, pole vaulting,diving, or dancing is difficult to a body which moves with efficiency. The same principles apply to all of these seemingly divergent activities.

Co-ordination is the ability to direct energy through two or more sequences of muscles at the same time either in unision or in counteraction as necessary for the desired action. This can be achieved only when the body has become so well trained any given action is achieved by kinetic response rather than thinking through the action and then transferring to muscular action. It is obvious that many times the mind interferes with co-ordination rather than aids in specialized action. Many times in teaching the dance I have been told by a pupil that he is lacking in co-ordination. A completely false statement in-so-far as his kintetic response, for immediately following such a statement he may walk across the room, talking as he does so and carrying a heavy parcel. The ability to achieve these actions was learned at too early an age for him to still remember the period of transference to kinetic response. Only those actions in a specialized field where he is conscious of the learning stage cause him any difficulty in coordination. It is true that he is making action in his accustomed field more tiring by using the wrong muscles for true efficiency, but he is basically not lacking in coordination. We rarely see a person, no matter what bad posture or however awkward, who takes other than an even pace in walking, who stumbles on stairs from lack of a kinetic sense of how high to lift or lower a leg to reach the next tread, or who crushes a glass or drops a heavy object in handling. Given these simple abilities, that person actually holds the potentialities for good carriage or posture, graceful or efficient movement, rhythm, and even complex coordination.

2. DANCE

The following experiences in the field of rhythm and music with mental patients is purely a statement of observations during actual working periods with mental patients. Owing to the fact that we have been under pressure because of the large number of patients, there can be no scientific approach to the subject. At no time has a comparison been made between groups having the benefit of rhythm and music against a control in having such an experience. Comparison has been made with a group before such experience and during the experience when sessions were being held. Owing to time limitations no statistical records have been kept.

The following will consist of observations made during my time spent at St. E. Hospital together with an explanation of the techniques used at that hospital. The past five years of work at St. E. in Washington D.C. was a fortunate period for experiencing the many difficult aspects of work with mental patients. During this period the changes that have occurred have given workers at the hospital a chance to develop in a much broader way than it would seem possible during almost any other period. We have seen the hospital change from an institute covering treatment over a long period of time to one in which pressure of time and the acute illness of military patients necessitated rapid work; and have then seen the hospital return to a more quiet institute again.

During this period one was able to view the differences between chronic illness and acute situation illnesses very clearly. In reviewing the past five years it would seem that it must have covered a much longer period because of the changing conditions within the hospital.

St. E. is a particularly fortunate hospital in which to work in a field parallel to that of the doctors, owing to the open mind of the hospital staff and the general feeling of cooperation between the medical and nursing staff and those working with other forms of therapy.

From the time I first started as a volunteer, working with selected groups, until the present with both selected and unselected groups, the hospital has been ready to give all help possible and to encourage any new ideas that had sound basis. For this reason, I feel fortunate in having been able, within the one hospital, to have had such a wide experience.

We have used music and rhythm for relaxation, stimulation of interest, group activity in varying types of wards, from the small special class on prescription from the doctors to the most intensely ill wards of overactive or depressed patients. The groups have varied from small ones of 8-10 patients to full ward coverage 40 or 60 patients.

We have used this method of approach in continuous daily sessions and in scattered classes given at intervals. We have used it in combination with choral and group singing, with painting, and preliminaries to psycho-drama sessions. It has been used for social poise, in teaching ballroom dancing, and in relaxation in conjunction with electric shock therapy. In other words, there has been an opportunity to use it in nearly all forms of possible hospital experience.

At no time has it ever been used other than as a means for group activity and for ward experience on a social level. We have found that it seems to be a means through which mental patients are able to tolerate and be tolerated by small groups. Thus, while under treatment, they are regaining and rebuilding experience while still within the hospital.

I wish to stress that this form of activity has been used as therapy only in the broadest sense of contact with patients and always on the conscious level.

3. THE USE OF DANCE IN WARD PROGRAMS

The mental hospital of today is turning its back more and more on the point of view of the past, which accepted the fact that many patients would require care in this setting for long periods of time. Today, everyone from the doctor in charge to the nursing assistant thinks of the hospital as a therapeutic community and there is only one goal for the patients, his return to the outside community.

In spite of this attitude, which creates a structure of the greatest use to the patients who are able to return to the community in a short time, there will be many patients who will continue in the community for longer periods as hospital citizens. Much of the hospital care for a considerable time will be devoted to these people. With a concentration of various forms of therapy being devoted to the rehabilitation of the patients who will be leaving, there are often fewer personnel and staff available for these where change occurs more slowly. Many patient activities with the more passive patients leave the leaders, whether nursing assistants or recreation workers, feeling that they are out of step with the more active parts of the institution. Patients often continue to show extreme lethargy over periods of time, no matter how earnestly and with how great enthusiasm the personnel work.

Since dance is an activity which will draw patients to it no matter how lethargic they may seem to be, I always feel that it is most useful with patients who find it difficult to participate with others, particularly in these activities where an acceptance of competition or verbalization is required and where demands from the outside for conformity are a tacit part of the session. Dance is based on movements of non-verbal communication and it is therefore a medium which meets the withdrawn patient with tools which are understandable to him.

I always have dance sessions in one of the buildings at Saint Elizabeths Hospital on an afternoon when movies are shown in the theater building. This session is open to any patients in the building who wish to attend. Although some people have not consented to go across the grounds to an undemanding activity, these same people will come to the dance room and the session can be geared to their needs and provides an outlet for them. There are usually fifteen or twenty patients who have resisted urging to go with the group and yet who can become involved in the music and movement session even though their intention had been to remain solitary and passive on their wards.

There are many places in a hospital where dance is useful in the same way. It is often as helpful to the personnel as to the patients. It is so easy to become accustomed to accepting refusals to participate in anything and the breach caused by the withdrawal of the personnel as well as the patients widens.

It must [illegible] us that dance sessions are useful to patients who are ov[illegible] have short spans of attention and consequent bursts of i[illegible] sessions furnish an acceptable medium for release of t[illegible]rgy and the possibility of functioning with other peo[illegible]

D[illegible] for building better coordination and a feeling of co[illegible] in the rehabilitation programs, but if I were cho[illegible] patients for whom it is most useful, I would list those [illegible]use frustration to the personnel through their lack of participation and ability to become personally involved.

An Outline for a Book on Dance Therapy

Marian never wrote a book. She did write an outline for one. Perhaps some of the prior notes were intended as an introduction to the contemplated book. If so it was as far as she got–to our loss.

INTRODUCTION

Will cover the general aspects of variety of experiences of the twenty five years at St. Elizabeth's and the different experiences at Chestnut Lodge.

The comparison between work with the sudden acute illness of the military and the difference between that work and that with civilians.

CHAPTER I

Approaches to mental patients and differences between that and the approach to so-called normal people.

Similarities, differences in working with mental patients and children.

Purpose and aims of rhythms in dance and music.

CHAPTER II

The purposes and aims with the convalescant, the methods of approach, the use of simplification, its correlation with psycho-drama and case work interviews.

Development of group interaction and group direction.

Use for stimulating interest in other forms of activities and in the world at large.

Development of interest in other patients and the beginnings of social awareness.

CHAPTER III

Dance with chronic patients.

The importance of its use within the hospital.

Importance of awareness that it is for the purpose of relaxation and stimulation of interest within a limited environment.

Need for lack of drive toward perfection.

Development of a group coordination within the hospital wards and recognition of the class continuing indefinitely without the possibility of great improvement or change.

The possibility of this being used for better ward spirit, brighter moments of integrating harmony, interest in other hospital activities, development of permanent friends within the hospital wards.

CHAPTER IV

Use with overactive patients of the acute type.

Need for acceptance of lack of concentration.

Excited and disoriented behavior.

Sudden changes of mood.

Acceptance of very strong antipathy and rejection.

Purpose and aims to enable patients to relate to one or two people or to small groups with confidence and without effort.

General purposes are relaxation and a few minutes of quiet.

Use of movement for getting rid of strong aggression.

CHAPTER V

Depressed patients.

Need for acceptance of quiet and inertia.

Dangers of lifting individuals or ward atmosphere too high in pitch.

Purpose is to bring about activities into the ward and a few minutes of lift ending with a change of mood toward the lighter and brighter.

Use of movement and group activity to bring about an awareness of reality and less absorption in patients' fantasies.

Dangers of entering into the patient's fantasy rather than bringing him out.

Methods of approach.

Meeting of the patient on his level and taking him with you.

Importance of lack of pressure.

Importance of quick movement from patient to patient.

Need for extreme simplicity and directness.

Need for awareness of patients without initiative to join, to indicate in some light manner, "Do you wish to join?"

Feeling of neglect.

CHAPTER VI

Music with catatonics.

Approach of patients.

Lack of discouragement.

Need of stability.

Constant awareness of his awareness in spite of no response.

Awareness of attempts on his part to communicate in pantomime.

Awareness of his moment of exhaustion and pressure of the presence of another person or persons.

Use of movement to make him willing to trust sufficiently to dare verbalize or speak.

The use of movement for relaxation for intake of food.

CHAPTER VII

Use of music with painting.

As a means to relaxation with convalescent patients.

Stimulation of former interests and new interests in music.

Stimulation of interest in study of music through enjoyment with a group with similar interests leading to possibility of such in the outside world.

Stimulation of discovery in patients when he is not alone in his interest of art forms.

The value of audience in creative arts where defeat had been met as an artist.

Awareness of interests in art having value.

CHAPTER VIII

Use of music and movement with electric shock.

Type of music used for resting, changes as they awaken.

Stimulation of conversation.

Stimulation of group conversation.

Use of rhythms and exercise following treatment.
Stimulation of intergroup activities and group coordination.
Stimulation of desire for activities in other directions.

CONCLUSION

Work running parallel rather than entering into without the physician or the social worker felt.

Development of poise, feeling self assurance and confidence as other methods of treating a psychosis immediately are being successfully achieved.

Bringing Dance Therapy to Israel

In July 1964 at the age of 67 Marian Chace took her first and only trip abroad. She went to Israel and in three short weeks did nothing less than establish dance therapy as a permanent part of the Israeli mental health professional team. Her trip was sponsored by the State Department and had the active support of Dr. Dale C. Cameron, then superintendent of Saint Elizabeths Hospital.

Nothing attests better to Marian's power to project the meaning of dance and its therapeutic potential than what she did in Israel. She did not speak the language and came from a different culture yet she moved patients and staff. Dalia Razin, who was Miss Chace's interpretor and guide on the trip described how after one session an old woman who was a patient in the hospital came up to her and said, "She brought love to us." And indeed she did.

Marian kept a journal on her trip. This in itself is unusual because she apparently did not record any other period of her life in such a detailed fashion. Her sharp eye missed nothing. She had time to be aware that each tree in the Jewish National Forest stood for someone who died in the holocaust, to make comments on the food in the kibbutz, and to record her reactions to the sessions she ran. This document is produced in its entirety. In addition there are copies of some of the newspaper stories written about her activities, and a letter to Dr. Cameron after her trip.

1. JOURNAL

July 11, 1964

I arrived in Tel Aviv, Israel on the evening of July 11. The plane had stopped at Rome where I changed from Pan-American to an El Al plane. This line has by far the most comfortable planes and the best service of any plane I was on. If I were travelling to the middle east again, I would want to travel by El Al, the Israeli air line.

I had my first experience of the very modern way of life of many of the people in Israel. While the structure was of white concrete which is used a great deal throughout the country, it might have been in the suburbs of New York or Washington. The floors were of tile for coolness, but the room was furnished with simple modern furniture, universal for all good hotels and inns, had air conditioning, excellent service and my balcony overlooked a lighted swimming pool and I could hear music from the night club.

The following morning I drove with Mr. Amiran, music director in the ministry of education and culture, who was responsible for my invitation, and who devoted the entire time I was there to seeing that the course went well and that I had every comfort and need taken care of. I also met the young dancer who was my interpreter and companion. She travelled with us as well as Mrs. Bucky who had accompanied me as an individual on the trip.

The road between Tel Aviv and Jerusalem is a wide well kept highway. The land is very flat and deserty except where irrigation makes the fields of vegetables and orchards very green and productive. On this road one begins to have the awareness of the mixture of the old and the new. There were many Arab villages which were like pictures one has seen which looked as though they had not been changed or renovated since Biblical times. The people wore Arab clothing, dirty and unkempt and here and there were Arabs in the fields helping on the farms. As we approached Jerusalem the hills began to appear and the temperature lost the humidity.

Again, the mixture. We stopped at a roadside stand which was near where Samson was born but which looked like a stand near Coney Island.

Then began a winding drive through the hills near Jerusalem. The people of Israel have done a fabulous job of planting trees by hand and the hills are becoming forested. One tree for every Jew killed in the German concentration camps. Here and there along the road as a reminder of the days of struggle were the burned tanks used in keeping the road open during the siege of Jerusalem. On the higher hills were old monasteries and everywhere small Arab villages, terraced gardens, vineyards and orchards being sprayed with enormous streams of water.

Traffic is heavy and there is a constant stream of travel between Jerusalem and Tel Aviv.

Jerusalem has a very beautiful skyline. It suddenly appears rising on the hills ahead. Jerusalem has many trees and has a unity in its appearance as all buildings, whether apartment buildings or private homes, are built of Jerusalem stone, a beautiful cream colored sand stone. At sunset the colors of rose and violet are overwhelming in beauty.

We went to the place where we stayed immediately. It was one of several flats where visiting teachers at the Rubin Academic of Music are housed.

It had a balcony overlooking a wide expanse of Jerusalem with a view of the university, the concert hall and the houses of the new Jerusalem. I shared the apartment with my interpreter companion. We were lucky to have a kitchen where we ate breakfast and many suppers. No matter how hot the day when I went home for a siesta the thick walls, tile floors and a strong breeze through the slatted window made it cool and restful.

The midday siesta is a necessity. Everything closes and people sleep from 1 to 4. The day starts at 7:30 and resumes after the siesta at 4. One works then until 7 or so.

After leaving the bags, I went to the Rubin Academie of Music to meet Dr. Dostrovsky, a very distinguished and warm person. The Academie is built around a patio with flowers and shaded by an old tree, left standing when it was built. The Academie is a very busy place where many courses in music and dance are given by visiting artists. There is so much eagerness for education, that people come from all over Israel and there are too many people in the classes.

My first impression of Israel was the mixture of the old and new in buildings, people and cultures. Here at the Rubin Academie of Music I gained my second impression of the drive for education which goes beyond an eagerness to learn. These impressions grew during my visit. I was also made aware of the warmth and openness of the people. I was welcomed and generously honored throughout my stay.

The first week was an orientation to Israel, both old and new places and people. I was so busy from morning to night, occasionally even during siesta time that I will perhaps not have the proper chronological sequence.

The first person I met away from the Rubin Academie, was Dr. Miller who heads the Ministry of Mental Health. Dr. Miller is a friend of Dr. Cameron and was very interested and hopeful that the dance therapy workshop would be useful. He gave support during my stay in many ways. In conversation he seems very aware of the psychiatric thinking outside of Israel as well as inside.

I also visited Professor Vinik, the head of the Talbieh Hospital, a mental hospital of 750 beds in the city of Jerusalem. They are working to keep patients out of the hospital as much as possible although many of them have readmissions at intervals. I met some of the patients, saw the wards where they lived, watched them working in the OT department, met some of the OT workers and talked with them about the structure of the program when I would bring the students to do sessions with them.

They have a day hospital similar to ours, use some drug therapy and a great deal of verbal group therapy. There were a few patients from the fanatic Jewish sects and a small number who were from the more oriental groups, but the majority seemed a cross section of the Jewish population of Jerusalem.

One evening was spent in listening to Israeli folk music, as I was uncertain of the response to the music I am accustomed to use, with the patients here.

We were fortunate to go to the home of a young builder and his wife who is a painter and musician. They had converted a stable in a lovely garden into their home. The many arches had been retained and it might have been in the Village in New York. They were formerly Americans but intend to live always in Israel. As with many people they seemed a part of both cultures. We even had apple pie and coffee as refreshment. Our hostess assured us she often served this. It was good to see the beautiful Israeli hand crafts in this home.

Since this was an extremely old stable, I had a feeling that it could be similar to the stable where Jesus was born. It belonged to that period and they had retained the original feeling.

These four days were also devoted to the sightseeing of any tourist. We drove through the narrow streets of the fanatic Jews and looked down the narrower alley streets where men in side curls and long black coats and women in heavy black clothing lived, shopped in crowded shops and performed their religious rites away from the other people of Jerusalem. Their places of worship are very beautiful, it is said. The buildings are obviously very old and have been there for a long time. If anyone offends them, they stone the offender as was done in early days. Consequently, they are left to go their own way.

During the first four days I visited a number of places in Jerusalem.

Ramat Rachel is a high hill on the outskirts of the city. Since there are many spots which are in the hands of the Arabs where one cannot go, the best one can do is to look from a high point. One of the things that is tragic is the number of these places. From Ramat Rachel one can see the road to Bethlehem and also the town itself in the rounded desert hills.

From this point, too, one can see the Dead Sea in the far distance and know that Arab outposts are out there.

Even in Jerusalem the wall keeps some of the places of antiquity from being actually visited. Here at some points where we came close to it we had to be careful not to stand with our heads above the wall for too long.

From the roof of the Notre Dame convent which is open to visitors we could see the old city of Jerusalem which could not be visited. But there was a wide panorama of viewing. Even the Wailing Wall of the Jews is denied to them.

We visited the beautiful new university buildings which has had to be built because the older university is in Arab hands and standing empty. Nothing could be more beautiful than these buildings and grounds. Again professors are excellent but the drive for education causes the classes to be very crowded.

The music concerts are very heavily attended. The concerts are long and no concession is made to make the latter part of a concert diverting and light. The people of Israel have more concentration than we have. My first concert was on Sunday, July 12. It was by the Israel Philharmonic Orchestra. It was all Beethoven.

Overture—Leonore #3

Concerto #3 for piano and orchestra

Symphony #5

The 2nd was choral group from all over.

The 3rd was a very heavy modern concert.

The 4th was Menuhin in chamber music.

The concert halls in both Jerusalem and Tel Aviv are very large—beautifully wood panelled and acoustically better than any I have been in in this country. The tickets are not expensive and the halls are crowded. Whether it is someone from one of the ministries or just a citizen, there seems to be no distinction made. The galleries outside the auditorium are wide and very alive during intermission and are all glass enclosed. The concert hall in Tel Aviv is next door to the Habima Theatre and the one in Jerusalem is on a high hill next to the university.

Two very exciting events were seeing the Chagall windows at the Hadassah Hospital and the Dead Sea Scrolls in an air conditioned vault at the University. A beautiful domed building with proper air conditions is being built for the Dead Sea scrolls. One very interesting afternoon was spent at the International Congress of OT at Kfar Shaul, a work hospital for chronically ill patients. There was very interesting OT work with goals, beautiful and creative painting and people in charge who seem to know what they are doing.

The new university has a very beautiful campus. The architecture of the buildings is simple and satisfying in line and the halls are wide with high ceilings which are restful and conducive to study. I understand that the professors are outstanding and the people spend much time in study.

On Thursday morning we left Jerusalem to drive to the north of Israel. We went through Tel Aviv, a busy city of modern buildings, filled with balconies, cylinders on the roofs for making use of the sun's rays for heating water, wide tree lined avenues and many people. American factories are everywhere. We drove up the coastline where we could see glimpses of the shoreline. The Mediterranean is very blue and as with any sea shore setting there was a continuous line of small villages of summer cottages. People go to the sea for weekends as much or more than we do. To the right were the desert hills and fields of green which were cultivated by irrigation and constant watering.

In the hills were landmarks of early Biblical times and the new clusters of houses in the Kibbutzim.

We passed through Haifa, which is a beautiful new city built on a high hill where the white houses are enclosed in beautiful gardens. High apartments and hotels dominate the tops of the hills.

We continued north where the hills become young mountains and finally arrived at the Kibbutz Mishmar-Haemek.

Our hostess was a delightful older woman who taught Dalcroze eurythmics and had lived at Mishmar-Haemek most of her adult life. Her rooms had very modern and simple, colorful furnishings with prints, ceramics and colorful draperies and rugs. Outside was a beautiful garden and a view of wide fields under cultivation. During the evening there was a gathering of a group of her friends with pleasant, stimulating conversation.

This kibbutz is old enough to have developed wide lawns, flower gardens, winding walks with trees and a general atmosphere of a summer resort.

Here we saw for the first time the children's houses where they are cared for by people assigned to this instead of the parents.

The rooms are cared for but are like dormitories. There are cubicles for the clothing of the children, common bathrooms and rooms for the recreation of the children. It was all fine if the children had been orphans or at schools from which they would go home. During the hours for the children to be with parents one could see mothers walking with the children or sitting on a lawn playing with them.

There were school buildings which were like schoolrooms anywhere, a delightful room for the Eurythmics and a large room in a separate building for music.

We ate dinner in a large room where everyone in the kibbutz eats at long tables where carts of food are wheeled around for rapid parcelling out of food. Whether dinner, supper or breakfast, the food is the same—cucumbers, tomatoes, strange cheeses like sour milk somewhat thickened, bread and strange mixtures of eggplant, hard boiled eggs and meat or fish—grapefruit juice and tea are the beverages.

People are assigned to cook, wash dishes and serve. Apparently people are not chosen for their ability to cook and the food which has been cooked is remarkably tasteless. The clattering noise and numbers of people at the long tables makes relaxed conversation difficult and people seem to be gathered for the purpose of eating quickly rather than sharing a social hour while eating.

People living in the kibbutzim now have time for cultural activities as well as hard work. There are concerts, folk dances and many other shared activities of this sort.

The work of the kibbutzim has changed from work in the fields to factory work. At Mishmar-Haemek they make the plastic dishes for planes and lamp shades of plastic for general sale.

The people living there seem dedicated to their loyalty to the kibbutz.

From here we travelled through the hills to a town on the Sea of Galilee called Tiberias. This is a very luxurious resort which might be anywhere.

Luxury hotels and houses which I understand are patronized by people from everywhere in the winter. The blue of the sea and the hills make it beautiful.

We also drove through Nazareth. It was too bad that we didn't have time to stop. But we did see the twisting narrow streets and old houses that looked as though they had been there since the days of Christ.

We then drove along the shore of the Sea of Galilee to Kibbutz Afikim which we used as headquarters for two days. It was on the Sea of Galilee which is called Lake Kinneret in Israel but in spite of this it was unbearably hot.

The people were very welcoming to us as they had been at Mishmar-Haemek. They lived in the same way, but it was larger and not as beautiful. They did have a beautiful amphitheater on the shore of the lake where many concerts with visiting artists as well as the members of the kibbutz are given.

In the morning we drove past River Jordan and up the shore of the Sea of Galilee to the glorious high mountains north of Galilee. The hills are rounded and from them you can look over miles of fertile valleys. We were told that nowhere is there the peace that seems to be there. Over the hill were Arabs always alert. However, we saw the Arabs only when we were in Jerusalem. But everywhere on the roads of Israel were both men and women soldiers going some place.

At the top of the mountains you come upon an old village built on the steep slopes of the mountain called Safed. Here a group of artists live where they feel they can paint. Their homes have the usual balconies and furnished roofs where you can see views that are overwhelming and beautiful.

In some of the narrow streets a group of Jewish philosophers live spending their lives in contemplation. They wear the long black coats, and twisted curls in front of their ears.

We went back to Kibbutz Afikim. In the evening we visited a newly uncovered floor of an ancient Jewish temple and spent the rest of the evening talking with people in the kibbutz, some of whom are involved in the life and some who questioned very much their way of life.

On Sunday we drove back to Jerusalem and my peaceful cool flat where I would live during the next three weeks of the workshop. My companion was a lovely young dancer who was my interpreter and who accompanied me nearly everywhere.

We drove across the mountains, through Haifa and along the Mediterranean to Tel Aviv and on to Jerusalem where we saw the sunset on the buildings of Jerusalem, so unforgettable.

On Monday morning I met the members of the group with whom I was going to work.

They were a group of 45 good looking eager young women who worked in various hospitals, schools and clinics from all over Israel. Some of them taught Dalcroze eurythmics, some were occupational therapists, some nurses and some psychologists. While many of them worked with groups of people none of them knew about group work as we know it.

The first week consisted of some lecturing and some working in the techniques of dance therapy. It was an exciting and moving experience to work with people who give their entire attentive concentration to listening and learning.

At the beginning the people were very restricted in their movements. This was a great deal from their training. They wanted to be told what to do in an ABC, 1, 2, 3 way, But a little bit at a time they absorbed the idea of relating movements to what is going on. A group began to form. At the beginning few people knew each other.

In addition to the lectures and practice in the movement of dance therapy the group had classes in dance, demonstrations of the way in which different teachers conduct classes in eurythmics.

Dr. Schossberger, the head of a work hospital called Kfar Shaul, gave classes in an understanding of the behavior patterns of mental patients.

We were fortunate, too, in having Dr. Vinik of the Talbieh Hospital and members of his staff attend the sessions and make comments.

Miss Yael Yoalit, who is in charge of the Occupational therapy program and training in Israel, attended nearly all. She acted as interpreter for me when someone was lecturing in Hebrew just as Dalia Razin, my interpreter, translated from my English to Hebrew for the group.

One interruption that was happening continually was a stream of reporters for interviews which were published in the newspapers of Jerusalem and Tel Aviv.

One exciting evening in the first week was the open lecture I gave to the people of Jerusalem. Because the professional people for the most part, have English as their second language, at least in understanding, I could speak without an interpreter. I spoke in the beautiful patio garden of the Rubin Academie to an audience of 150 or 200 people. Again, it was an eager group who listened intently and asked many good questions. I was fortunate to have Dr. Vinik introduce my talk and Dr. Miller, the head of the Ministry of Mental Health, summarize the talk. It was a stimulating and heart warming evening. Dr. Miller was supportive of all of the things that happened and is interested in continuing the use of dance therapy throughout Israel. He stated after the lecture that I had conducted it with communication in body action. He also stated that he had rarely seen such a responsive audience in Jerusalem.

On Friday evening I had dinner at the home of Dr. Schossberger with his family and Dr. Vinik. It was a quiet evening with pleasant and stimulating conversation as well as their opportunity to get acquainted with me. They were the psychiatrists in charge of the hospitals where the group would work with the patients.

On Saturday I was the guest of honor at a formal luncheon at the home of some of the VIP's of Jerusalem where I talked about dance therapy. It was very pleasant but not stimulating.

Saturday evening I attended an informal, unofficial party of some of the old citizens of Jerusalem who had had a lot to do with Israel in the early days of its independence.

Sunday was the first session with patients at the Talbieh Hospital. This is a 750 bed hospital with a very well trained staff. The patients are not kept in the hospital continuously but are at home as much as possible. While some tranquilizers are used the treatment consists of group therapy, activities, both occupational and recreation therapy, work assignments, including the care of a large garden. While there is not a large number of psychiatrists and social workers, there are enough for what seems to be a well integrated program with team work. Comparatively small numbers of patients are under one administrator. The groups for the dance sessions were chosen by the administrators.

The sessions were held in a large rather plain room. We worked with three groups of patients. They were composed of both men and women and were not separated as to degree of illness. I would say that the proportion of European patients in the groups was similar to that seen in the city of Jerusalem. The group consisted also of a mixture of withdrawn, depressed and over active people.

It was necessary to discard my rule that all observers must be participant observers. Everyone on the professional staff who could possibly do so, including the nurses and occupational therapists, attended the sessions. There were also a number of people from outside of the hospital involved in the mental hygiene programs who also attended. The guests coupled with using only a few at a time from the group I was teaching caused an audience of fifty or sixty people at all times. I was surprised that the sessions went well, even though the audience was seated at the end of the room.

I was also surprised at how the patients' actions and reactions showed little difference from those in the United States. It was very obvious that emotions are similar although cultural patterns are different. My language difficulty made no appreciable difficulty for them. Relationships were being made through body action and tone of voice. Specific words were not important.

Occasionally there was something that had to be treated in a different way, but which could be handled easily. In one group there was a young man from one of the fanatic religious groups. After moving by himself for a time, he joined the circle. However, he entered between two women.

Since he is not supposed to touch women, we had two men stand on either side—, so that he would not feel guilty afterwards. He continued to cut through the circle at intervals and seemed to be relaxed. While he didn't verbalize very much, by the third session, he was greeting people and chatting for a moment. One thing that helped is that he is accustomed to dancing in a circle with men at his religious services.

Another young man who wore his cap at all times participated not only in his own session each day but came back for the others. At the end of the second day he returned after the others had left and sang not religious, but secular songs for us with apparent great joy.

One group of patients in verbal therapy were too relaxed, according to their therapist, to use their hour for verbalizing. They stated that they had expressed their feelings fully in the dance session.

It was interesting to watch the changes in the group during the four days we were there with sessions.

The first day there was a tentative acceptance of us—, with more freedom of action toward the end of the sessions. Faces lighted up and there was a small amount of verbalization with the beginnings of relationships with individuals in the working group they greeted us with welcome on the second day and the same was true on the third day.

However, the group was much more quiet on the fourth day. Apparently, they had learned that this was our last day to be with them. At the end of the session they presented us with a bouquet of flowers which they had picked from their own garden.

Israeli music was played at first, but they were involved with the activity and were responsive for only short intervals and then would respond with the usual involvement when the waltz, polka or other clear and simple records were played.

The nurses and doctors reported a reflection of more interest and initiative on the wards after sessions. Patients who had not been included in the sessions expressed a feeling of having been left out. A number of these people were permitted by the staff to attend on the last day.

Many individual incidents occurred which were very moving and I am sure had a value of carry-over into other situations. As usual, the patients who seemed to derive the most benefit, and who were the most involved, were the ones who were speaking only a little or not at all, particularly those who had language difficulties. Many of the people who were in the training group showed great sensitivity in reaching out to the more regressed patients. We had reached many of the patients with friendship, but it was sad that there could not be an immediate continuation.

A number of the psychiatrists, psychologists and nurses attended sessions of the trainee group a few times and one of the occupational therapists was a member of the training group.

On Thursday of this week we went to a very interesting hospital under the administration of Dr. Schossberger called Kfar Shaul.

The setting is unusual and beautiful from an interesting point of view. It is situated on a hill close to Jerusalem with a wide view from most spots. Unlike the Talbieh Hospital, it is a collection of small buildings which are very ancient. It was originally an Arab village which has been converted into a well equipped living place for patients who will spend a considerable time here.

One building is for a group of patients who have privileges of going into town to work and use this building to return to at the end of the day. Only a house mother is there and the patients care for the quarters themselves. They even cook some of the meals. The house mother lives with them. They have made the rooms as attractive as possible. It is similar in its setting to many halfway houses in the United States even to self government meetings.

One of the buildings is a canteen, again largely cared for by the patients.

The dining room is a large cheerful room and the O. T. shop is also a cheerful place. Throughout Kfar Shaul one is impressed with the thought in the organization and the dedication of the well trained staff. Again, one of the O. T. workers was a member of the training group and others of the staff attended sessions at intervals.

The O. T. program is a well thought out and organized one. The patients are encouraged to do creative things while they are too sick to work for perfection, but as they improve they have a program of making useful objects which can be sold, and a sale is held once a year. Some of the chairs, fabrics, pottery and other objects were very beautiful and one wished it were the time of the year when one could buy them.

The art work too was good and is on a graduated program.

We were able to see the structure of the program because of the exhibit which had been arranged for the International O. T. conference which had just been held there. Dr. Schossberger gave us time in explaining why they did certain things in the art therapy program and when they moved into more structured work.

A great deal of time is devoted at Kfar Shaul to the gardening and the flowers are beautiful. In both the Talbieh Hospital and at Kfar Shaul the patients take great pride in the gardens.

Not all of the Kfar Shaul is an open hospital and a great deal of purely custodial care is what some of the patients experience. There is an attempt throughout, however, to involve the patients in useful work projects within the limits of their abilities at the time. As with all places it does not reach everyone.

After the visit to Kfar Shaul was over, I left rapidly for Tel Aviv to give a lecture on dance therapy to the professional people in that area.

There was an interested and interesting audience and it was good to meet the people who live in the modern city of Tel Aviv. A group went to one of the sidewalk cafes, which is a part of the life in Tel Aviv.

The following morning, Friday, I had a one day dance therapy workshop for eighty of the physical education teachers who work in the schools throughout Israel. The day consisted of lecturing and conducting sessions with them. No one intended to use the techniques as such but wished to learn new viewpoints to add to their own work. As with the group in Jerusalem they were all interested in learning, and there was no problem in holding the attention.

Friday evening I was fortunate again in attending a home musical evening. People who are finished musicians often gather together to share with one another the music they love. Although this was the Sabbath evening they apparently felt that an evening of this sort was appropriate. Among the groups of people I met I found nowhere the feeling that all activity must stop on the Sabbath. They accept the stopping of public transportation, but everyone uses private cars and cabs to move about. I was staying at a resort hotel with a swimming pool and gardens. On the Sabbath, Saturday, the pool and gardens at Rabat Aviv are open to the public and many families have picnics together and use the pool. Hundreds go to the shore of the Mediterranean for swimming, again in family groups. Often on the roads you will see groups of hikers going up into the hills for a one day holiday. Israel works on a 6 day week so that if people did not use the Sabbath for these activities, there would be no time for it.

I had counted on a day of rest for this Sabbath for myself but instead I went into Tel Aviv to tape a talk on dance therapy in the morning and then had a very pleasant chat with a member of the physical education teachers' organization. In the evening I attended a concert at the concert hall in Tel Aviv. This was a concert by Menuhin and his sister with others supporting them. It was chamber music throughout. In spite of the size of the concert hall, the acoustics are so good that it was most enjoyable. I like the auditorium in Jerusalem better. It is much less elaborate than the one in Tel Aviv. However, there is an interesting group of buildings in beautiful grounds, a library, the concert hall and the building which houses the Habima Theatre, which I regretted not having time to attend.

Early Sunday morning we drove back to Jerusalem for the first session at Kfar Shaul.

I had asked for patients who were either not ready or not willing to participate in any of the program at Kfar Shaul. We were involved at first with two groups, one of women and one of men. Many of the patients were mute and at the beginning were solitary and very resistant to participation. But as members of the training group approached them individually while those who were ready to move together were moving in a circle, little by little they joined in the activity. Two or three very hostile people were able to express this hostility and then were among the most active participants.

One woman who had readily joined the women's group at first sat sullenly in her seat on the last day. I was told that she had had an experience on her ward that was upsetting to her. However, when the men's group arrived she took on the role of an assistant and participated throughout the session.

These sessions were most difficult because of the large number of staff as well as outside visitors who were watching. We were helped by the interest and cooperation of the O. T. personnel.

One man remained both mute and motionless for quite a period of time on the first day but one of the training group sat with him quietly and gradually he began to move and eventually joined the circle.

Each session used strong vigorous movement across the floor for a part of the session and some of the men even seemed to enjoy jumping and running before the end of a session. This in spite of the fact that they had been passive or resistive at the beginning.

Part of the way in which they showed us courtesy was by serving us punch and cakes between sessions. This is characteristic of all the people of Israel. Always the inevitable fruit juice and cakes when you are visiting.

My last day of sessions was at a children's center. This could only be in the nature of a demonstration of what might be possible. This is a well equipped school with a large and well trained staff. However, we worked in a very small room with five or six children at a time. There was such a large audience that it was overwhelming in this space, as the audience took up more space than we had to work in. The children responded amazingly under the circumstances. I am sure that this was because the group leaders participated with us. The American cultural attache visited this session.

The visits to the hospitals involved only the mornings, but the group of trainees had classes in various activities from 3 or 4 to 5 and then they met with me for an hour or more to discuss and work on problems that had come up at the sessions.

My last week was a very hectic one. I tried to do all of the things that had not been done. One day I was entertained at luncheon by the mayor and others in the government of Jerusalem, another day I talked at noon to the staff of the new psychiatric unit at the Hadassah Hospital. At present they have only sixteen short term patients in psychotherapy. The Hadassah Hospital is a large, very well equipped General Hospital which is new and very beautiful. It stands on a large hill some distance from Jerusalem and dominates the landscape. There is a small pavillion attached to the main building which houses the Chagall windows which have been given to the Hadassah Hospital.

Another day I had lunch with our cultural attache, Mr. Henry. This week I did not have the usual siesta that everyone takes.

The evenings were just as crowded. There was a concert at the Rubin Academie. I spent a quiet evening with one of the members of the group in the interesting converted Arabian stable. The group gave me a wonderful party, with folk singing, dancing and a general festival of warmth. This was also attended by some of the doctors and others in charge of various things connected with the course. Another evening was spent at the home of a member of the ministry of culture. I packed and left for Tel-Aviv, arriving in time for two hours of shopping on Friday before the stores closed.

Then dinner at the home of Mr. Amiran who was responsible for everything and where I was too weary to be really gracious. Finally a day of rest on Saturday; my first since I had landed in Israel, and on to the plane for Athens and points west.

2. Translated From Ha-Aretz of July 22nd, 1964

Reprinted courtesy of *Ha-Aretz*.

"Visitors' Galley"

DANCE AND MUSIC AS MENTAL TREATMENT

This is the third year that the Rubin Academy of Music in Jerusalem is holding its summer course program for musicians and performing artists. During July and August intensive courses are held in music and dance. Teachers and advanced students are occupied in their work all year. Performing artists do not have a sabbatical, and for most there are no scholarships. Younger people in these fields do not have the opportunity to increase their knowledge and broaden their scope by studying at renowned studios abroad and with the most famous teachers and instructors from abroad to Israel. As the Academy's director, Mrs. Yosheved Dostrovsky, puts it: "This is a meeting with renowned musicians and teachers who contribute to the nurturing and development of art." Thus, for example, we had here two years ago the famous dancer, Martha Graham, and other great artists. It is very difficult to bring such personalities to Jerusalem during the year, but in summer it is possible, and there are some who have returned, such as one of America's outstanding pianists, Mrs. Nadia Reisenberg.

This year, in addition to the courses in music and dance, there will be a special and unusual course—dance therapy—under the direction of Miss Marian Chace who is head of the department of Music And Dance Therapy at St. Elizabeth's Hospital, Washington, D.C., which has 7500 patients. Her method of dance therapy has been recognized by doctors and others in the profession in the U.S. Her many articles on her method which have appeared in scientific publications have earned her an award from the U.S. government for her service to the American nation. She represents her country as an "ambassadress" without a diplomatic passport.

This woman, well on in years, radiates a feeling of faith to her listeners, and her love of Man, and with the strength of her faith, she has succeeded in working miracles with hundreds of patients with whom she has worked. Israel is the first country Miss Chace has ever visited, but in her own country she has conducted dozens of courses of instruction in her method. Generally her pupils are the nurses who specialize in treatment of mental patients, but also teachers of rhythmics and dance as Miss Chace's method endeavours to release from mental depression healthy persons as well, and not only those who reach mental hospitals.

Her object is the establishing of communication between the person with his fellow-man; to shatter the walls of his silence, where he has isolated himself behind barriers of fear of his surroundings.

Marian Chace herself arrived at her present profession through the dance. For many years she was a dancer and choreographer, a teacher in the Denishawn School. She also had her own dance company. In 1942 she began to devote herself more to the development of her method of dance therapy and was invited to join the staff of St. Elizabeths.

Miss Chace's method includes no magic or hypnotism, but only a deep insight, using the same natural means as those means whereby a person himself tries to make contact with others. "In movement one can express contact", she explains. For example, when the patient is entirely cut off from his surroundings, he has visions, and hovers in other worlds; he isolates himself and hides from society, does not respond to ordinary means of communication, such as speech. In such a case, Miss Chace will seat herself beside the patient entirely without movement exactly as he is. Then she will start soft music and slowly begin to move one leg, for example. After a while the patient will do likewise. She will then proceed to move her arm, or some other part of her body, and the patient will again imitate her. This establishes the first contact between them.

"No man wants to be alone", says Miss Chace, and in this law of humanity is the hidden basis for success. The next time the patient meets her, they already have something in common—without having exchanged a word. Gradually, she draws him in to take part in some sort of group activity. "And so I smash the barrier of silence. Movement is what gives the spark of life to the patient''. In other words, movement gives him courage and gives him back his self-confidence.

In the many years of experience in her work, Miss Chace has perfected her method to adapt it to the varied cases, as each one is different. Miss Chaces' method is not a final cure in itself, but a link in the general process of treatment in a hospital and depends on the work of the staff of physicians. The method is not a ''medicine'', but only an instrument, says Miss Chace, but its use rests on the belief that it is possible to rehabilitate mental patients.

The course will include practical work at Talbieh Hospital and Kfar Shaul in cooperation with the Department of Mental Health of the Ministry of Health, and the Department of Music Education of Ministry of Education & Culture.

3. Translated from MAARIV of July 23rd, 1964

Reprinted courtesy of *Maariv*.

> MENTAL PATIENTS DANCE TO HEALTH Marian Chace, dance teacher of Washington, D.C. engaged in ''treatment by the aid of dance'' comes to Israel to teach her method.
>
> by Nili Friedlander.

The blue eyes of Marian Chace have seen thousands of those isolated, withdrawn from all normal contact with their surroundings, safely hidden behind the walls of mental institutions— and as she speaks of those human beings, this silver-haired woman sounds impressibly sober: ''Within ourselves we are all alone,'' she says, and in her eyes one sees softness, understanding, and deep sympathy. Perhaps not all is lost; even the silence of the alone-ness is sometimes broken. She believes, because she has heard with her own ears.

Once there was a small group of patients waiting for her in a room. She entered quietly and started the phonograph. To the strains of a waltz, she began to move, and they followed her. Gradually, as they overcame their hesitation and fear, they began to speak to each other. They conversed. Communication was established!

It is now 20 years that Miss Marian Chace has been occupied with dance therapy and she has developed it from its beginnings to a complete method. Before starting in this direction, she was a dancer and dance teacher. Even then she noticed that many who came to her studio did not necessarily want to be dancers. By body movement, which is the most spontaneous method of self-expression, they sought to solve their problems. Nevertheless, even after she was invited to teach dance at St.

Elizabeths Hospital in Washington, D.C., as she was not yet convinced that she could effect actual cures through dance lessons, she hesitated to devote herself entirely to this work.

Today she is the head of the Department of Music and Dance Therapy in the hospital in the capital. In dance she sees a way of reaching the patients. She usually works with them in groups of 15-20, not with individuals, "because that is the natural way. Each person alone, but we all have to get used to living among people." In this field she is considered the world authority.

All those who presently belong in this field of dance therapy are her pupils who have adopted her method which she has spread by means of lectures to doctors, dance teachers, nurses of mental patients, and by her articles in medical journals and in dance publications. She received an award from the U.S. Government in recognition for her service to the nation. She is now in Israel to conduct the first course of this kind here which opened at the beginning of this week at the Rubin Academy of Music in Jerusalem.

This is the first time that she has ever left her native country. "I've simply never had the time," she explains.

Her "discoverer" was the composer, Emanuel Amiran, Directing Supervisor of Music Education in the Ministry of Education & Culture. Mr. Amiran visited in the U.S. on a UNESCO Fellowship to see the institutions of music education in the U.S.A. He had the opportunity to visit St. Elizabeths at that time. He saw patients, sitting about, as motionless as stones. Miss Chace entered the room and began to dance. "I had read that she does wonders," said Mr. Amiran. "One of the patients came up to me and took me to dance a tango—which I won't forget for the rest of my life."

On his return to Israel, Mr. Amiran got in touch with Dr. Louis Miller, director of the Department of Mental Health, and Prof. Winnick, head of Talbieh Mental Hospital. The director of the Rubin Academy was very enthusiastic and agreed to include a course in Dance Therapy in its summer course program which began this week.

Forty-five nurses, physiotherapists, and teachers of rhythmics and dance are participating in the course. After attending lectures by Miss Chace and Dr. Schussberger, director of Kfar Shaul, the students will also do practical work at Talbieh Hospital. Other lectures will be given by Hassia Levy-Agron, Mr. Kalev, Dr. A. Friedman-Witkower, and Dalia Razin. Mrs. Razin will be assistant to Miss Chace, and will carry on the work of dance therapy, the basis of which will be obtained from this course. Mrs. Razin has already had some previous experience in this field while studying in the U.S. and Switzerland (mainly in dance therapy for backward, disturbed, and handicapped children.)

Miss Chace will give two additional lectures to doctors and nurses, in

Jerusalem on July 23rd and in Tel Aviv on July 30th. On the following day, she has kindly consented to hold a one-day seminar for physical culture instructers which will take place at the Seminar Hakibbutzim in Tel Aviv.

4. Translation from LAMERCHAV, July 24, 1964

Reprinted courtesy of *Lamerchav*.

DANCE EFFECTS COMMUNICATION by Ami Shamir

Can a person be cured by means of dance? A strange question but the answer is even stranger: Yes. Miss Marian Chace, a gray-haired, noble-looking woman of 67, believes this with all her heart. She has come here from the United States to teach the basic principles of her original method to a number of nurses and therapists.

Marian Chace had never left the U.S. and her visit to Israel is the first such trip she has made in her life, although word of her doctrine has reached far and wide. Her travels were generally to the "far countries" of the mind, or to be more exact, to the depths of disturbed minds, so geography played a very minor part in her life.

Actually, she is a dancer. For 30 years she devoted herself to the dance as a dancer, choreographer, and director of a well-known dance company. As a dancer she noticed the "magic" powers of dance and the great satisfaction that her pupils derived from it. "I saw that even people who did not intend to become professional dancers took dancing and became very enthusiastic, and I came to the conclusion that herein lies something very important which should be developed". And indeed she did. "The idea grew by itself," she says, her gray eyes twinkling. "I asked psychiatrists and doctors to send me their patients who refuse to talk. I want to try to make them respond by means of dance. It turned out that my premise was correct: patients found that dance was a more efficient means of communication than talking, which they rejected."

This was a beginning for her method which she afterwards developed when in 1942 she was invited by St. Elizabeth's Hospital, which has 7500 patients, to head the department of Dance Therapy—the first to be opened in the U.S.A.

The principles of her method have been published in her articles in medical and educational journals.

"Non-verbal communication between human beings," says Miss Chace, "existed before speech and in the world of words in which we live—crammed full of the spoken word, the broadcast word, the projected word, and the printed word—these have buried the pure means of expression by movement which was predominant earlier in the development of human society." Expression by movement reveals a truer expression of feelings. Movement is not only a means of individual expression but also a pure means of social communication, and a wonderful medium to express symbols, ideas, emotions; and feelings. Movement expresses moods, and opposed to the spoken word, it always bears the imprint of sincerity; it is impossible to "deceive" in movement as with words. Movement calms and absorbs pain—a thing known to every mother as she rocks her baby.

From this we have practical conclusions about people who are mentally disturbed. In a mental patient the power of speech loses much of its efficiency. The mental patient locks himself in a world of silence, the walls of which cannot be breached by means of speech. The only way to reach him is by non-verbal expression, namely, music and dance. Miss Chace tried this and succeeded. The worse the condition of the patient, the greater the success of her method: using dance to penetrate the thick wall of defense and make the first opening towards normal relations between them and others.

How does this work in actual practice? Miss Chace brings a group of chosen patients to a room provided with a record-player and records. After a warming-up period in which she allows the patients to choose the music they want, she forms a circle which starts to move to the strains of a waltz. The movements at first are simple but after a while some of the participants show an inclination to more intricate movements. She then turns over the leadership of the "lesson" to them, and it passes from one to the other, and the therapist only lends encouragement. After a while the mood improves and several of the participants even show a desire to speak. Here and there some laughter is heard. Patients who feel at ease encourage the reluctant ones. In the next step, the patients break off into little groups or individually to improvise by themselves. Here are created spontaneous dances as the dancers give reign to their feelings. The "lesson" ends in listening to soft music and vocal discussion wherein a wide range of expression to the emotions is given.

The choice of music is suited to the prevailing mood of the group. For patients with depression she plays waltzes, polkas, squaredances, etc. But for patients who tend to be excitable, lively fast music quickly changes to quiet and soothing music. Preferred works are Bach suites and Debussy preludes.

Dance Releases

The results of these "lessons" are amazing. "Dance", says Mrian Chace, "releases the participants from their tensions which frequently appears as extreme tightening of the muscles, aggressiveness, and so on."

After an hour's dancing the patients start asking the therapist or one another: "Who are you? Where are you from?" This first achievement is renewal of communication; social contact has been made. Of course this is only the first step in the therapy and not the cure itself. Dance does not work miracles; it only "breaks the ice" and shatters the walls of isolation, and so makes it possible to continue treatment by therapy of accepted means.

These reservations are all her own, but not those of others in the profession who have recognized her wonderful achievements and bestowed upon her an award, the highest decoration granted by the Health Department of the Department of Health, Education & Welfare of the U.S.A. Within the last 20 years her work has aroused great interest not only in America but abroad. Experts from Sweden, France and Holland have asked her for advice and guidance, and invited her to set up an organization of dance therapists similar to the American association of music therapy, of which she is an active member. But Miss Chace has declined all these requests the only invitation she accepted was to give her course in Israel.

The "godfather" of this project was Mr. Emanuel Amiran, directing supervisor of Music Education in the Ministry of Education & Culture who met Miss Chace while in the U.S. on a UNESCO fellowship. Mr. Amiran was so impressed by her personality, her dedication and her work that he decided to make every effort to bring her to Israel. There is great therapeutic power concealed in music and dance, says Mr. Amiran, which we do not exploit at all. I realized this when I saw Marian Chace at work in St. Elizabeths Hospital in Washington, D.C. I immediately thought of the possibilities of applying her method for our schools and mental hospitals. He thereupon spoke to Dr. Louis Miller, head of the Department of mental health, and Prof. Winnick, director of the Talbieh Mental Hospital in Jerusalem, who responded enthusiastically. There remained only the problem of financing her trip and the organizing of the first course in dance therapy. The Rubin Academy of Music in Jerusalem came to the rescue by agreeing to take the responsibility for this. (The Academy includes a department in dance in its syllabus).

Dr. Dale Cameron, director of St. Elizabeths Hospital and Miss Chace's employer, approved her visit to Israel, as he had visited Israel a few years ago and saw our great need in the field of mental health.

Training of Teachers in Her Method.

It is most interesting to note the great response that resulted when registration for the course was opened. It seems that Marian Chace's original idea fired the imaginations of Israelis no less than it had that of the Americans. In a very short time 45 applicants—nurses, therapists, teachers of rhythmics, and even one man—signed up for the course which started this week. The course will continue until the 7th of August, and will include lectures in psychology, psychiatry, and other allied subjects, as well as practical work at Talbieh Hospital.

The object is to prepare local experts who will be able to carry on the work after Miss Chace returns to America and to spread the idea of dance therapy in educational work and in the mental hospitals. Israel's serious problems in this field cry out for additional means and new ideas, and Mr. Amiran did a good deed, indeed, by intervening in a matter which is not really in his province, and hopes now that the seed that was sown will bear fruit.

Dalis Razin is certain of this. She is a graduate of the Music College in Jerusalem who studied in Switzerland and the U.S. music therapy in the treatment of deaf-mute and disturbed children. Dalia is at present acting as chief assistant to Miss Chace in Israel and she is very much impressed with the visitor's personality whose whole heart and soul are in her work. Dalia is convinced that a great deal of good can be done with the help of Miss Chace's system.

And what does our guest think of us? "I was a little afraid before I came", she admits. "I heard so much about your cultural and scientific accomplishments that I was uncertain how you would receive my modest contribution. And in addition there was the question of language. But apparently my fears were groundless. The human material in the course is excellent and the desire to learn is great".

We asked Miss Chace why her method has not received international recognition after it has been in use for over 20 years. Her answer: That is the fate of all new ideas, and what are 20 years in comparison with the eternity of man's soul?

5. Translated from DAVAR, August 7th, 1964

Reprinted courtesy of *Davar*.

COURSE IN DANCE THERAPY ENDS
CONTACT ESTABLISHED BY MEANS OF DANCE

A special course for dance therapists ended this week in Jerusalem. The course, of three weeks duration, was under the supervision of E. Amiran, Directing Supervisor of Music Eduction in the Ministry of Education & Culture, and under the auspices of the Ministry of Eduction, the Ministry of Health, and the Rubin Academy of Music.

Forty-five participated in the course, among them teachers of rhythmics, physiotherapists, psychologists, and dance teachers. Instructor of the course was Miss Marian Chace of the United States, originator of the method in whch she is engaged at St. Elizabeth's Hospital, Washington, D.C.

The purpose of the course, held here for the first time, was to teach the principles of the method intended primarily for the treatment of mental patients, to give those who wish to work at this confidence in working with mental patients, and to accustom them to feel the patients' reactions and to learn from those reactions.

Success in the U.S.

The method of dance therapy has achieved wide success in the U.S.A. and has even reached Europe. The method is based on establishing contact with the patient who is completely withdrawn within himself and removed from his surroundings, by means of body movement with background music. As Miss Chace says, Speech is often used to conceal feelings, whereas body movement reveals and bares feelings. The background music creates an atmosphere in which the patient can express himself in movement. Movement results in a release from tension, and is an expression and proof that the patient wants to make contact with his surroundings. The doctor attending the patient can then take advantage of this situation to continue with his treatment.

Astounding Results Here

During the course the participants did practical work at Talbieh Hospital and at Kfar Shaul, and even in these sessions Miss Chace achieved astonishing results. According to the therapist in charge, there were some unbelievable instances.

One patient, for example, had absolutely no contact with people. In the beginning, when the background music started and other patients began to move, he did not react at all. Little by little, he began to make small, stiff movements, but without joining the rest of the group. After a while, when all were sitting in a circle and joining hands, the rhythm caught him, too, and he started to move while sitting, and much to the surprise of those attending him, at the end of the session he joined in the group activity. The following day, he was more relaxed and joined in immediately at the beginning of the session, his face more animated.

These astounding results have aroused interest in the medical profession. It is expected that many of the participants in the course will apply this method to practical work in various hospitals.

6. Letter to Dr. Dale Cameron

STATE OF ISRAEL

Ministry of Education & Culture
Department of Music Education

84 Hashmonaim Street
Tel Aviv

August 11, 1964

Dr. Dale C. Cameron, Superintendent
St. Elizabeths Hospital
Washington, D.C. 20032

Dear Dr. Cameron,

Now at the close of Miss Chace's 3-week course in dance therapy I am very happy to report that the success of the course exceeded our highest expectations.

I have no words with which to thank you for allowing this truly remarkable woman to come to us and shed the light of her inspiring personality.

From the enclosed clipping from the JERUSALEM POST and the translations from the Hebrew press you can see that the course caused not a ripple, but a wave, of interest. Her astonishing results in making contact with the patients, so well-known to you, greatly impressed not only the participants in the course, but the leading people in mental health: Dr. Louis Miller, head of the Department of Mental Health, Prof. Winnick, head of Talbieh Hospital, Dr. Schussberger, head of Kfar Shaul, Dr. Assael of Talbieh, and others. These people will give their utmost support to continuing Miss Chace's method in their institutions. In Miss Chace's opinion, many of the 45 participants in the course will be able to carry on with what they have learned from her.

As supervisor of music education I see in her method a very serious educational force which can be transferred to kindergartens and schools of normal pupils as well. In fact, if it were possible to give these basic principles to the general public it would be of great value in helping people who are too shy and too reserved to be able to express themselves and to release their tensions.

In my letter to Mr. I. Dandolo of UNESCO, Paris, from whom I received the grant to visit the United States, I mentioned that it would be worthwhile to take advantage of Miss Chace's unique method, if possible, and spread it throughout the world, so that everyone can benefit from this wonderful woman's understanding and sympathetic approach which brings a more human relation between people.

At the close of the course, many of the participants were moved to tears at parting from their instructor who had so endeared herself to them.

Marian Chace has left her imprint and will be long remembered in Israel, and for this I thank you again.

Yours very sincerely,

E. Amiran-Pougatchov
Directing Supervisor of
Music Education

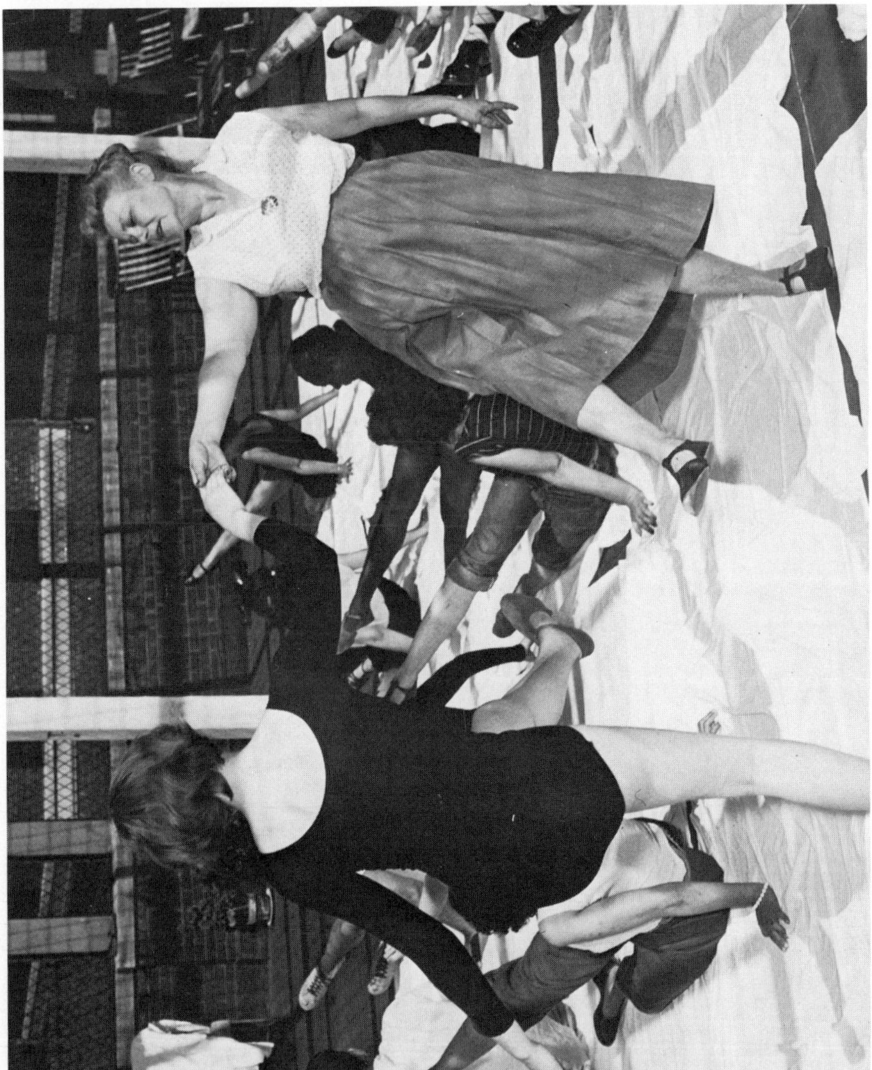

PART II

PUBLISHED MATERIALS

Rhythm in Movement as Used in Saint Elizabeth's Hospital

Reprinted courtesy of Beacon House Inc. from *Group Psychotherapy: A Symposium*. Edited by J. L. Moreno. Beacon, New York: Beacon House, Inc., 1945. Pp. 243-245.

There is a tendency on the part of certain patients in a mental hospital to remain motionless and mute for long periods of time, or to move about restlessly and avoiding contact with other people. Rarely, when left to themselves, do they gather for group activities. One method used at St. Elizabeth's Hospital for the encouragement of group activity is through classes in rhythmic movement.

The writer of this article was asked to try an experimental class in dance rhythm with a group of women patients in July in 1943, under the auspices of the American Red Cross which conducts an extensive but atypical recreation program at the hospital under the direction of the medical staff. Her previous experience in correcting behavior patterns of children who were anti-social, and in aiding adults with special personality problems, not sufficiently pronounced to need psychiatric care, together with several years of training at the Denishawn School of the Dance and as a member of their concert company and teaching staff, furnished a background for the use of dance movement as a medium for group activity with people not pre-disposed to cooperative action with each other.

During the past three years the number of classes has grown so that they now cover a large part of the hospital. Many forms of dance are used on both men's and women's wards. They are graded according to the degree of illness or convalescence of the patients rather than on the perfection of technique achieved by the individuals in a class. A patient starts in some class when he first arrives at the hospital, whether he is over-active or confused, catatonic or depressed, and he may continue in successive classes until he leaves here.

At first, only those movements which can be understood, by visual presentation or the sense or touch are asked of him. Later through gradual steps, he becomes able to participate in a formal class in which stress is laid upon posture, efficiency of action and a conscious group feeling.

On the women's wards and on the wards where catatonic male patients are cared for, rhythmic exercise is used, but on the balance of the men's wards the accent is placed upon social dancing. It has been found that many of the men patients at this hospital feel ill at ease on the ballroom floor, and consequently fail to take an active part in large gatherings of this nature. Through the class for the practice of ballroom steps, and the social hours with men too sick to leave their wards, many patients have gained confidence in meeting new people socially by the time they progress to open wards.

All classes, whatever the degree of illness of the patients in that particular ward, are conducted in a circular formation. Hands can be held around a circle, and a group unity achieved with patients who are too confused to remain attentive without the support of the group. It is possible in this formation to hold together as many as twenty-five catatonic patients. In this group they will do rhythmic exercises together—swings or arms and legs, stretching and limbering movements, bending and twisting actions, and even jumps and trots. These people will stay together while hands are held around a circle but will scatter into the far corners of the room to resume their static postures as soon as hands are dropped.

On an over-active ward, group rhythm in a circle is the only form which will enable the patients to feel free to join the activity for the few minutes that they are able to stay with a group in the midst of their own rapid, restless dance patternings. The circle often seems to act as a magnet, drawing them toward it, when they are too absorbed to speak or to join a formal class if they were asked to do do. This seems to be a satisfying grouping to the patients themselves, for they will form the circle for themselves, even when they are very confused, if the group leader fails to do so at the expected moment. While, on a convalescent ward, they will already have grouped into this formation before the dance director joins them.

By using a method of holding the patients together long enough to achieve a group rhythm, they are able to move about the room or to stretch long-unused muscles and gain a purely physical reaction of loss of tension with a definite improvement in body posture and co-ordination, no matter how confused and distrubed they may be emotionally. A growing self-confidence and ease of physical action keeps pace with their convalescence from their emotional disturbances. As the doctors prepare them to meet people more easily, they have acquired better equipment with which to do so. Poise and a lack of individual self-consciousness has many times been demonstrated by the convalescent patients at the hospital by the ease with which they have taken part in style shows and demonstration classes for large audiences.

The dance director who expects to stimulate strong, simplified but unified movement in confused, restless, mute or motionless patients must be willing to be flexible in her approach, and have acquired a technique to meet their varying moods, in other words, play the role of "auxiliary-ego" at all times in her contact with mental patients. The mute drama of the dance may at any point develop into a psychodrama.

It is essential that when a session starts on a ward, where excited action is in progress, that the leader meet this with movements of equal force. In contrast when she enters a ward where the patients are almost totally lacking in the initiative necessary to move about or talk, she must be able to speak and move as quietly as the occupants of this ward. From these widely separated extremes the muscular action of the patients is carried by means of infinite varieties of group rhythms, to a mean degree of activity, and a quiet ward is left with movement that is pleasant but not too rapid, while an over-active group will have been led to a few minutes of quiet.

In doing this, sensitivity to action initiated by members of the class is an essential and in this way the form of the sessions does not grow into a rigid pattern, but can support and aid the patients in the group.

Not only must the leader be in sympathetic union with the moods of the patients, but the music used must also be in their own tempo and the color of the tones be those with which they are compatible. Whether an assistant plays a piano or gramophone recordings, this holds true. Again as with the rhythmic action and the approach of the dance leader, the music starts rapidly and loudly on an active ward, or softly and with no distraction on a depressed ward, and from these points it moves toward music that is strong rhythmically but not exciting. On the wards where catatonic patients are in the majority, men who have shown no inclination to talk, will sing as they walk in rhythm together to such songs as "I've been working on the railroad", and "Tavern in the Town" and afterwards gather around the piano and to sway together and sing songs of Stephen Foster. On the post-shock ward, men who are just coming out of the coma will sit up in bed with a smile as the songs of our folk culture are played and sung. Movement about the room, physical action in harmony with a group, and relaxation of tension are the aims of rhythm in movement as used at Saint Elizabeth's Hospital, rather than technical achievement as at a dance school.

Dance Therapy at St. Elizabeths

Reprinted courtnesy of the National Association for Mental Health, Inc., from *The Psychiatric Aide,* 8 (September, 1951), pp. 3-4.

Moving together with music breaks down barriers between patients and employees.

Everyone responds to rhythmic sound more actively than by merely hearing it. While one is listening, his body tends to feel a desire to move in rhythm to the sound. This rhythmic action in unison with others results in a feeling of well being, relaxation and good fellowship. Even primitive man understood that a group of people moving together gained a feeling of more strength and security than any one individual could feel alone. It was with this attitude, and with this premise, that dance was first introduced in the wards at St. Elizabeths Hospital about six years ago.

Many patients participate in the various groups from the time they enter the hospital until they leave. During the period of their stay at the hospital there is some form of group dancing or exercise in which they are able to take part, regardless of the degree of their illness.

The feeling that he is completely alone seems to be one of the overwhelming problems of the mental patient. On a ward of very depressed patients, one sees in extreme form this feeling of inadequacy and aloneness, separation from the group, and inability to believe in oneself or one's neighbor. Here the people are almost completely dependent upon the nurses and aides for every need; yet the very nature of their illness makes this situation difficult for them to accept.

In starting our dance sessions on the depressed ward, the leader purposely enters the ward very slowly, almost indifferently, her shoulders relaxed, and wheels the phonograph into place without haste. She then sits beside one of the patients as quietly as those around her, until one of the patients asks if she may start the music. This is the leader's cue to begin the program.

Everyone of us has had the experience of having some piece of music recall a painful or joyful episode. This is just as true for mental patients. For example, many pieces of music are disturbing to them. Curiously enough, one type that is not is waltz music. It may bore some people, but it does not disturb them. Consequently, waltzes are always used here to begin the session.

Waltzing in couples is done for about five minutes, since that is a familiar way of dancing in our culture. Then a circle is formed, and the part of the session is begun that brings smiles to faces, more freedom of movement and conversation. The movements consist of arm, leg and body swings; steps easy to follow by watching; walking, running, body stretches, and exercises for relaxing muscles. None of the rhythmic movements require previous training, as the stress is placed on the unison rhythmic action for the purpose of feeling relaxed together. Gradually the music is speeded up, and often polkas and square dances are used to finish the session.

For a long time now, the nurses and aides have accepted the dance program. During the dance session, not only is the leader of the program moving with the patients, but also as many of the nurses and aides as can be spared from other duties. It is not unusual to see one of them comb some patient's hair, then join the dance circle with her, and later go on to an easy conversation or game of cards with her. A relationship has been strengthened that seems to make other activities easier.

I have often been asked whether dancing together later causes difficulties between the staff and the patients, when a nurse or aide must use a firm attitude for the good of the patient. Since dancing is as common to many people as talking, listening or walking, this form of relationship does not seem to confuse the patient as to the respective roles of patients and staff within the hospital.

On those wards where people are so quick in their change of mood that they are fairly unpredictable, the session starts with rapid music and movement. Gradually the music and activity become more quiet, and the session ends with people in restful postures as they listen to soft music for awhile.

As patients become convalescent, they come to the dance room for sessions in body control and coordination through exercises in the modern dance. The student nurses here are a part of the class. Since they are in class for only a few sessions, the majority of the patients are more proficient at the exercises than the student nurses. The patient-members of the class take greater pains to reassure the student and make her feel comfortable about this, and so a ready give-and-take is established. It is difficult, after this, not to see the members of the dance group as people rather than as patients.

So much of the possibility of a mental patient's return to health is dependent upon establishing a basis for mutual understanding with those who are closely associated with him. Many factors in a mental hospital which seem necessary—the carrying of keys by the staff, and not by the patients; giving of orders, and obedience to them; freedom on one hand, and lack of it on the other—cause natural barriers between personnel and patients. It seems as difficult for the staff to see patients as people, as it does for the patients to see members of the staff as other than in a position of authority over them. The dance sessions seem to be a meeting ground where these barriers are less obvious than in many situations, and where understanding of each other as people may develop more freely.

This will happen, of course, only if the hospital aide is able to lay aside her attitude of authority and participate actively in the session on an equal basis with the patients. I believe that this will strengthen rather than weaken the relationship in their daily roles.

Opening Doors Through Dance

Reprinted courtesy of *Journal of the American Association for Health, Physical Education, and Recreation*, 23 (March, 1952), pp. 10-11, 34, 39. Now *Journal of Health, Physical Education, and Recreation*.

Dance helps patients come back to reality at St. Elizabeths Hospital for mental diseases

Man has made use of art forms—painting, writing, music, drama, and dance—as a means of communicating his inner feeling about himself and his environment, since the beginning of history and probably before that. Dance as an expression is recognized as the earliest art form—even before music.

Why Dance Was Introduced

With the premise that dance is a basic form of emotional expression, dance was first introduced on the wards of St. Elizabeths Hospital for mental diseases, Washington, D. C., about six years go. Many patients participate in the dance groups from the time they enter the hospital until they leave. During their stay, there is some form of group dancing or exercise in which all are able to take part, regardless of the degree of their illness.

Mental patients feel very much alone. They feel an overwhelming inadequacy in their ability to communicate with others. Many times, their feeling becomes so intense that they rarely speak and then briefly.

Dance Among Depressed Patients

This separation from the group and inability to believe in oneself or one's neighbor is very apparent on a ward of depressed patients, who tend to remain apart from one another, sitting or standing alone for many hours at a time, lost in preoccupation with their own thoughts. Conversation is almost totally non-existent among these patients. Occasionally a nurse or aide will be able to hold the interest of one of them for a short while, or a group of patients who are feeling somewhat better will carry on a game of cards with the help of a recreation worker. Even reading and handwork are difficult for these people.

It is on this ward that one begins to understand why primitive tribes ascribe "magic" powers to rhythmic action in unison. As John Martin, dance critic of the *New York Times*, says "When we see a body undergoing muscular exertion we are naturally inclined to feel it in our own musculatures. . . . .this leads naturally to actually dancing in a ring with him, executing the same steps that he is executing."

Effect on the Patients

I have many times seen a patient, who was so withdrawn from the life about him that he was unable to talk, eat, or care for himself, be attracted to a circle of people doing rhythmic action together and be able to participate with them. Occasionally, the closeness of the unison dancing will be too much for such a patient, but he will be able to dance by himself with the support of the circle doing a unison rhythmic dance around him. The group participation gives him a feeling of confidence in himself that he seems unable to find alone.

Since this happens only when the patients are dancing in a circular formation, the dance sessions on this ward are always conducted so that a circle is formed. While there is a great dependence here on the leader to sustain the rhythm, just as there is dependence on the nursing staff for daily care, leadership does not remain entirely with her in this formation but can shift to various members of the group for short periods.

Requests for particular kinds of music will be made; conversation, laughter, and stronger body action will develop. For a short time preoccupation with distressing thoughts and isolation from the group have been laid aside and the process of re-socialization, which is a part of any hospital program, has then begun for some individuals.

How Dancing Is Done

The dancing on this ward is always done to music in waltz time at the beginning of any session. Everyone of us has had the experience of having some piece of music recall a painful or joyful episode. This is just as true for mental patients. Curiously, the waltz may bore some people, but it does not disturb them.

The leader first enters the ward quietly, almost sadly, wheels the phonograph into place, and sits beside some patient without even speaking unless the patient speaks first. In a moment someone goes to the phonograph with a request to play it and the session begins. Waltzing in couples is done for about five minutes, since that way of dancing is familiar in our culture. Then a circle is formed and the part of the session is begun that brings smiles to faces, more freedom of movement, and conversation.

The movements consist of arm, leg, and body swings; steps easy to follow by watching; walking; running; body stretches; and exercises for relaxing the muscles. None of the rhythmic movements require previous training, as the stress is placed on the rhythmic action in unison for the purpose of feeling relaxed together. Gradually the music is speeded up, and often polkas and square dances are used to finish the session.

The nurses and aides help with all of the dance sessions in the hospital and they often join the circle, bringing with them patients who are particularly withdrawn. Much of the possibility of a mental patient's return to health is dependent upon establishing a basis for mutual understanding with those who are closely associated with him. The dance sessions seem to be a meeting ground where the patients develop understanding of each other as people more freely than in many situations in a hospital setting.

Watching Is Also Active

Some patients are unable to participate actively in the dance sessions at first. However, even the passive participation of watching seems to be more active than one realizes, because many patients respond to the rhythmic action that they are seeing and the rhythmic sound that they are hearing.

One day, after Miss X had watched the rhythmic circle for some weeks, she finally participated actively. I made the error of telling her that I was happy that she could now be with us. She was very hurt and asked me if I failed to recognize her. I assured her that I knew her well. "Then how can you say that?" she asked, "I have been with you for weeks." I next made matters worse by saying, "I mean you were able to dance with us today." Again, she had the same hurt expression, saying, "But I have been doing that, too, while I watched. I am stronger now, that is all." At last I said, "Of course, I should have known." She helped me to remember always that the spectators are feeling the rhythm in their own musculatures and by so doing feel a part of the group.

Some patients are able to play the phonograph for the group before they are able to join actively in the rhythm circle. They will establish this as their self-appointed task, and, I am sure, feel as much a part of the group as those who are dancing.

Restlessness Expressed in Dance

Some patients in mental hospitals have very rapid changes of mood. Although they are not entirely cut off from conversation with others, it is difficult for others to follow their thought sequence, as their speech is influenced by their quickly changing moods. Just as their speech is rapid and difficult to follow in sequence, so are their movements restless and ever changing. These patients are always giving expression to their feelings with their bodies. When music is played, their response to it is very exciting. They are able to express their feelings in dance movement or in dramatic forms that are easily understood. They need no encouragement from a leader.

Miss Y was in a hospital where dancing was not a part of the program. She felt compelled to dance when music played, but the nursing staff would feel that she was becoming too excited and needed to be relaxed with hydrotherapy. Consequently, she was always torn between her need to dance and the outcome if she did. She felt that there was no one to understand what she was saying with her dance.

However, at St. Elizabeths Hospital, when one goes to a ward where people feel this need, one always sees some of the patients dancing. For a long time, I made the mistake of believing that some were trained concert dancers.

Today I realize that in the excitement of their illness these patients are able to dance with the freedom that we must spend time in study to achieve—and then not so effectively.

Forms of Participation

Although they do not need encouragement to dance, they do need a leader to use this dance pattern with others. Again, the circular formation enables many of these patients to dance with others for short periods of time. In addition to aiding the feeling of unity in a group, the circular formation also has other advantages, especially for those people whose attention span is very short. Participants can join the circle for a short time and then leave to dance by themselves or watch and later rejoin the group with no interruption to the group activity. During a session with patients who dance spontaneously, one sees circles of three, or six, or eight people moving together and then breaking apart only to form again in other combinations or go scattering apart to dance individually and then back together again.

On this ward, the music used is rapid and sharp in character at the beginning of the dance session. As time passes, the tempo is slowed until quiet chamber music is played, for listening purposes only, at the end of the session. This alone would be restful to these patients who seem to feel a need to be restless in their activities. They are able to rest for a short time after they have had an opportunity to give vent to excited action in a constructive way. On this ward, too, one may participate in dances of destruction and despair as well as gaiety and omnipotence, but all of them danced in a way that would cause any dancer to be excitedly sympathetic for their directness and originality in movement, since these people are able to speak so eloquently with their dancing.

As patients move on to convalescent wards they attend sessions in the dance studio in their own building. Here they learn body control as it is taught in dance sessions in schools anywhere. Also, as in dance sessions outside of a hospital, the more adept help those who need it and the group which had its beginnings on the wards of sicker patients becomes more aware of its members.

Is Dancing a Cure?

The question is often asked as to whether dancing is a "cure." This is not the function of dance therapy. It is one of the ways in which people who are mentally ill can be with one another without too much fear of defeat. This in itself is relaxing, quite aside from the effects of body exercise. It is one of the ways in which patients can again begin to feel themselves a definite part of a group and so begin, in a small way, to function again in society.

Physiological Aspects

Reprinted courtesy of the National Association for Music Therapy, Inc., from *Music Therapy*, 2 (1952), pp. 63-67.

In speaking of the physical aspects of personal gratification through music, I naturally will speak principally of the dance. In the majority of the world, it would be inconceivable to separate the two; anyway, their relationship is a basic one. Does it really matter whether one considers the individual as adapting himself in rhythmic body action to music or sound played by someone else, or whether one considers the feeling of the individual making that tonal or rhythmic pattern on an instrument while his musculatures throughout respond? Both people are feeling the release from rhythmic tonal sound that has been experienced by man from the beginning of history in all parts of the world. There is, to my knowledge, no group of people which has not had its own music and its own dance-forms as a part of its culture.

I believe that it was not accident that caused primitive man to make use of music and dance (or rhythmic action) for the purposes of both worship and solidifying group-feeling in a community. It was not accident that the "magic" of the medicine man (or spiritual leader) was performed through rituals of chanting and body action.

Unfortunately, in our own culture we are not so aware of the potency of rhythmic actions and music, as we should be. We relegate the enjoyment of making music and dance to especially talented men and women who perform in a concert hall, where a large audience sits in silence attempting to remain absolutely motionless and giving vent to their desire to move only at those moments of pause by coughs, fluttering of programs and shifting of positions, which makes the hall sound for a moment as though a sudden restless wind had entered and passed through—leaving sudden stillness in its wake. Not so in the majority of the world, where group music and dance is part of the living, daily activity of the people.

Basic dance gives a more specific feeling of release, I believe, than the making of music on an instrument, as in addition to the universal response to rhythmic sound, people express their emotions through psychomotor tensions. Dr. Plant states: "The child is quickly made to realize his position of security. We are rather sure that the earliest transmissions of this sentiment are through the psychomotor tensions." Therefore, in the dance, the individual makes use of both of these means for emotional release.

If one ever felt that rhythmic sound and action were intellectual pursuits, divorced from the feeling of people, one would have only to visit a mental hospital to become aware that this is a fallacy. Here is every direction where people are living in their emotions, (or as the psychiatrist says, "Acting out"), one sees an almost universal response to rhythmic sound. Here, too, where behavior patterns are on an individual level and not that of the group, where behavior is more "unpredictable" than is usual outside of the hospital, or more stereotyped than the majority of us feel is necessary for safety, response to music has quite other meanings in terms of feeling from our own, or perhaps than we are willing to acknowledge.

Music and rhythmic action in therapy, then, should take advantage of this universal response of people. Those of us who are working in hospitals in this field, are working in no artificial medium, but a most real one. We are working in a medium which belongs to every living person. I feel very strongly that we should beware of this trap into which it is so easy to fall and which is fostered by "*our culture*," namely, that the arts are mainly for the specially gifted to use. We are not using the art to develop technically proficient performers, but to present to people (and, I mean people, not patients), a tool which is really their own to use.

I never like to speak entirely from my own feeling about music and dance when I am speaking of it in terms of therapy. I am merely the person creating a favorable situation for others to make use of the dance—if they so wish. For this reason, and because it is only fair for those people to whom it is so important, I always tell the group at St. Elizabeths Hospital that I am going to talk about the dance, and ask what they feel about it. Always I get many responses, which are incorporated into what I say. Once when this happened, a patient, who had danced a great deal but had never spoken, suddenly opened her eyes wide and said:

"Wait—you have not said the only important thing—'For a moment we live!' " . . . There was a little silence and then, responses from all. "Of course, that's it. She said what I feel too."

Could there be a closer, more important physical satisfaction to the individual than to "live" for a moment, to feel warm, free and most important, responsive and at ease?

Also, as I have just stated, there is so much importance given to this response by the patient involved, that I would be impertinent to even attempt to say what he felt. I always preface my request for a statement from anyone who wishes to make one by stating that I will be speaking from my own feelings about music and rhythmic movement, but that it would be impossible for me to more than speak of my feeling about his feelings, and so it would be preferable if he could tell me what to say.

This time, prior to coming here, I added that I was speaking on the subject of personal gratification in the physical area. The response gave me enough material to write indefinitely, as well as to take even greater care in the future that, as few of the people as possible with whom I am working feel unable to make use of music for their own needs of the moment.

I spoke earlier of the feeling of security being transmitted to the child through psychomotor tensions. Conversely, the feeling of insecurity is evident in the psychomotor tensions while extreme blocking of movement occurs. I have seen too many withdrawn, mute patients able to join a group of people through rhythmic sound or movement, to doubt the power of this form of the arts.

The responses of patients who are at the present time making use of music, while they are at the hospital, gave much more importance and significance to what they felt they gained, than I would dare to do!

One flatly stated the one word "Essential," another, "Like nourishment to the body," then added, "but, of course to the soul too, at the same time. We need both."

From another: "From infancy children should have it."

Out of this came a number of answers: "Recreates energy, rekindles energy," and, very important to someone who is usually very scattered and unsure of quite who she is: "Dancing and music coordinate mind and body"—and again in this area of thought: "Dancing limbers muscles literally and figuratively."

Because these remarks speak so directly of the feelings of the patients concerned and because they are so much clearer than many people are able to express, I wish to emphasize that they all come from people who are in an acute phase of mental illness, and, who for the most part verbalize very little about anything at all. I believe that the feelings expressed here have to do with the gratification of feeling the bodies alive, energetic and momentarily at ease—not only with themselves, but with others experiencing similar feelings.

One incident following a dance session illustrates this feeling of security as against insecurity in the group very well. We have been participating in a dance session where people had been working together easily and very rhythmically for an hour or thereabouts. Suddenly, at its close, one of the women, who had been working hard all morning, turned to me and, with intense anger in her voice and gestures, screamed at me: "You are too late with all this! How *dare* you deny to me all this from my infancy on, and now when it is too late, show me what life can be . . . how *dare* you?" I must add that after this outburst she returned to her ward quietly and for the remainder of her stay in the hospital, which was a matter of a few weeks, attended all possible sessions.

Sometimes this awareness of self, which is to me an important physical satisfaction, comes from one form of music, sometimes another . . . I remember distinctly one young service man, particularly, who first felt this when his fingers found a piano keyboard and he made sound at random. He crawled up from a curled heap on the floor and found the keyboard by way of the knee of the pianist sitting at the instrument. This young man happened to be a fine musician, but it would have been just as important to him had he not been. I have seen other patients first able to make sound again in an old song from childhood sung with others. Once sound has been made in song and the satisfaction of hearing has been felt, it is a short transition from there to conversation with those about him.

Whatever means a patient uses for participation with others, whether it is singing in a group, playing instruments in a rhythm band, or an elaborate orchestra, moving in rhythmic action with others or verbal conversation, it seems to afford him an active relief to get away from feelings he experiences while he is alone and isolated from others. The patients themselves, again, express this feeling in these terms:

"It gives me a feeling of belonging."

"You are with the group."

"It teaches you cooperation with others."

"I never learned to be with other people. I was never taught as an infant."

So many times the dance activity is related to what they feel they lacked in infancy and as a small child, and comes into their expression of the feeling of well being in the dance sessions at the hospital as contrast.

I have not spoken of the convalescent patient who feels satisfaction again, or for the first time—in achieving mastery of a musical instrument or body control in dance. Naturally, this is also therapy. Confidence in one's ability, satisfaction in technical mastery of one's physical equipment, is always therapy, wherever in the world it is achieved. But, it is dangerous to the individual I believe, in a mental hospital. He has so many mechanisms for shutting himself away from others, that again we who are using music as therapy should be sure that in developing a performer who will do credit to our teaching, we are not filling some of our *own* needs to the detriment of the patient. He must have spent many hours away from others in developing that technical ability. "Alone with his music" can become as much of a defense and as much of a "walking away" as anything else. To me, the therapeutic physical satisfaction comes from the awareness of *self* and *others* at the same moment, while participating in some form of tonal harmony.

Again I will quote from patients' expressions of their ability to make use of participation in a music activity for their own needs:

"Music and rhythm are outlets for the emotions."

"It fits every mood."

"Music feeds our soul."

"It breaks the ice in our feelings."

"Music helps us to express feelings."

"It relaxes and soothes."

I wonder if you have noticed two things about their own statements of their feelings. One is the frequency of comparing music and rhythm to food which they need for nourishment, and, the other is to the bridge it makes for communication with others. One statement is as frequently made as the other. Actually, both lie in the area of physical satisfaction,—gratification, first of all, for one must have a feeling of self, an energetic self, before one can reach out to others.

When we teach in the world at large, our end product is some art form of music or dance and our goal is development in the physical area of enjoyment and technical achievement. In the mental hospital, music is our tool to help the patient gain joy in the awareness of himself—accepting his role as a participant in some musical or rhythmic activity *with* or *for* others.

Techniques for the Use of Dance as a Group Therapy

Reprinted courtesy of the National Association for Music Therapy, Inc., from *Music Therapy*, 3 (1953), pp. 62-67.

In the world at large, people working in the arts have one of two goals toward which they are aiming, broadly speaking. The first of these is the use of an art form as a means for the communication of ideas or feelings from the artist to an audience. The second is the stimulation of young students and the supplying of the tools to them for building their artisanship. In both instances, the artist is working either with a sympathetic audience or with students who are able to externalize their feelings. All of these people have many tools for communication, many ways of relating to those about them. Consequently, the attention of all concerned in these interchanges of feelings or ideas can be concentrated within the framework of a specific art form.

The moment at which one steps within the walls of a mental hospital this setting changes. The people living within these walls are able to externalize their emotions either very unsatisfactorily to themselves or in ways that are difficult to understand. In addition, they have found their relationships throughout life either disappointing, frightening, or frustrating since direct communication is largely blocked for them. Thus, the leader of a group working here must necessarily shift his point of view from that of the teacher of technical forms in the arts to that of a group leader, using his particular art form as a tool for release of emotions or communication.

This is especially true of dance for hospitalized mental patients. An individual may play a musical instrument alone or in a group, gaining a great deal of satisfaction emotionally from both experiences. Painting and writing are rarely group experiences in the creative stages, both forms of art, as a rule, sharing with others the completed work rather than the work in composition. Dance, on the other hand, requires from the beginning that it be a shared experience for its full enjoyment. Even finished performers prefer attending or teaching classes rather than working alone. Only in composing a solo dance with the idea of performance will they dance alone.

The most widely accepted form of dance for our culture, ballroom or social dancing, is a part of the recreation program of any mental hospital, as it is in the majority of educational institutions. It is a form of entertainment to which patients look forward eagerly. In many places volunteer workers teach the basic steps to those interested. However, for the most part, these sessions are held in a central hall. Only those people who are able to manage with large groups for a fairly long period of time and with little supervision are permitted to attend. It is surprising, when the activity is social dancing, how many patients this includes.

However, this same activity could be taken to the wards of the hospital for those patients who are still too sick to participate in a large group. Here on the ward are people too shy to meet the demands of a fast moving social situation. Some of them have had painful experiences throughout their lives when called upon to relate to strangers or casual acquaintances immediately and on their own initiative. These same people, when well enough to attend the large hospital functions, will be found sitting back and watching as they have done all their lives while the more outgoing people make use of the opportunity for participation. Their patterns of adjustment to this sort of situation are unchanged and, except through accident, they will return to the world outside with the same role of watchers.

When a program of ballroom dancing is taken to these wards, confidence in the social situation, as such, can move parallel to other forms of therapy. Understanding of himself is undertaken with the help of the doctor, individually or in a group, manipulative skills are improved in the occupational therapy department, new ways of living closely with people are learned in the ward situation. Too often, though, many patients still find themselves lonely when others are having fun at a purely social gathering.

These ward programs, to be effective, must be undertaken with a change of point of view from the usual teaching goals. It is too easy to fall into the trap of teaching people more efficiency in ballroom dance forms and to concentrate one's interest as a leader on people who need little help in the social situation. They are the people who are in the center of whatever activity is taking place, either on or off the ward. However, if the goal is shifted toward furthering general movement in the ward, toward relaxation, and toward spontaneous group activity, before the session is over a beginning may have been made for some individual to feel more at ease in his casual associations. Some value can result from these sessions whether the leaders are trained personnel, interested members of the nursing staff, or volunteers from outside of the hospital, provided the goal for the session is the drawing into the group of the withdrawn person on the sidelines.

The session will probably, in its general form, follow any class in ballroom dancing anywhere, in or out of a hospital, with perhaps only one or two rather basic differences. In teaching, as such, the speed of the classwork is directed toward the upper half of the class. In the hospital, it seems to draw more people into the group if it is directed toward the lower half. The efficient patients can take care of themselves (they already have) and the speed will not frighten the slowed-up patient as it so often has in the past. The second difference is that of stimulating independent action away from the leader. It is better for the leader to follow leads and choices of music and steps, with the trend of the session coming from the group, rather than to achieve a well-organized class where the leader plays an authoritarian role. If the leader can sincerely feel that more has been achieved by some very shy person wishing to choose a particular record from the stack than by everyone in the room following her exactly, the dance session has probably helped someone to be, at least temporarily, more relaxed.

Modern or rhythmic dance sessions have much more value for mental patients than ballroom dance sessions. The social dance forms are exactly what they purpose to be, a means for helping an individual to achieve more ease in a casual situation. Modern dance, on the contrary, aids in several more important ways. Since it is a form of the dance which encourages the use of the entire body rather than the feet alone, it involves the patient in more basic feelings. The leader, for this reason, needs more experience in dance action and group leadership, and more knowledge of the behavior patterns of hospitalized patients. One of the problems of the mental patient is his feeling of unreality. This has a definite reflection in his body as well as in his emotions. His posture may be as good as it ever was, his action may be as efficient, but he doesn't feel that it is. Many times, of course, this is apparent in relaxed posture and lack of energy. He frequently eliminates himself from athletic contests because of his feeling of inevitable failure. In the same way, calisthenics seem overwhelmingly demanding in energy. However, many mental patients will accept some form of modern dance action, either on an individual or a group basis. Occasionally, they will be observers while getting acquainted, but later will be drawn into the action.

Music is an important factor in this ability of the patient to make use of rhythmic or modern dance action when many activities are impossible for him. It carries the patient and helps him to use his body action without too great strain. The melody and rhythm in the music together with the rhythmic action of the people about him draw him in almost before he is aware that he is participating with the group. If the dance action is taking place in a circular formation, he feels a great deal of support from the group. As John Martin states in describing tribal dancing, "In primitive societies spectators watching a dancer are frequently drawn first into beating a drum for him and then into actually dancing in a ring with him, executing the same steps that he is executing." If you substitute "choosing a record" or "dancing his own steps" for "beating a drum for him" you will have what happens in most dance sessions in a mental hospital. As in the sessions of ballroom dancing, the goal of the leader has been changed from that of the teacher to that of a catalyst for action. The leader is interested in giving support to patients as they feel their bodies moving in rhythm, for their own satisfaction, rather than in teaching complications of technical steps and actions to them. Conversely, at the moment that the dance leader shifts his goal from stimulating body action natural to the patient to teaching elaborate dance forms, he restricts the patient rather than aids him in emotional release or confidence in his own body action.

I have found sessions in contemporary dance most successful where the session started with totally free dance by patients who naturally make use of a dance form for expression of emotion, through unison movement in a circle, to spontaneous dancing singly, in small groups, and, finally, back to the large circle of unison movement. The leader should be spontaneous enough to transfer leadership to various members of the group, picking up the movements and translating them for the group. In this way the personnel leader remains a member of the group rather than assuming the authoritarian role of teacher. When a session is conducted in this way, it is surprising how many patients will make requests for help in improving body posture and action. A by-product of the sessions is more confidence for individuals in their own body action, which, in turn, helps them to relate to others. As one patient expressed this feeling,

"When the ice is broken and I can feel myself whole, then I can be with other people." Each dance leader will use, from his own technical background, those skills he has developed as tools in helping others to have confidence in their own emotional expressions, rather than in building highly adept dancers in a particular school of movement. I cannot stress too often the importance of this shift in point of view.

Any dance session should have sufficient freedom to permit an individual to dance by himself without feeling that he is disrupting the group activity. Often a patient cannot accept the close proximity, at the moment, of unison movement with others. If he can feel free to dance by himself with support from the group action, he will first dance outside of the circle, then within it, and finally, as part of the circle of patients. The feeling of sufficient freedom to do this will come from the structure of the group activity. Lack of rigidity, the leader's partricipation as a group member, with the accent on free expression rather than on absolute conformity to a predetermined structure for the session, will achieve this result.

It is, of course, advisable, when possible, to have trained leaders in any recreation program, but there are many hospital situations where recreation workers, as such, are either totally lacking or limited in number. Certainly, even in situations where aides are often called upon to furnish help in the activity for the patients, some form of dance as a ward activity may be used. They are often helpful as assistants, and many could be developed into leaders of dance sessions. In those hospitals where volunteers are, in the main, leaders in recreation, many could use dance as a tool as well as the accepted handcrafts, music, or games. Since modern dance has become a part of the curriculum of many colleges and universities, there are many people in almost any community who have had basic training in this form of dance. If they have received the training to be of value to the hospital in other forms of recreation, they are capable of using this tool for help.

In the ideal situation where a recreation worker can be assigned to dance as an adjunctive ward therapy he can be an extremely useful person. Where this is possible many patients will be found able to participate in groups who otherwise would be sitting alone, motionless, disrupting more structured activities, or compulsively knitting or playing solitaire.

Dance therapy essentially makes use of people's natural kinesthetic response to musical rhythm. Out of this can be structured sessions which are satisfying to many people, ranging from the area of social ease to the more basic fulfillment of emotional release and relating to others.

[Following the explanation, Miss Chace, assisted by six VA hospital staff members, demonstrated the techniques of dance therapy as outlined above with acutely ill psychotic patients in a simulated hospital situation: (1) with a group of withdrawn patients; and (2) with a group of overactive patients. Miss Chace's observations regarding this demonstration follow.]

All modes of nonverbal communication, by the very fact that they are nonverbal, are difficult to talk about. The translation from a nonverbal to a verbal mode of expression causes both a feeling of inadequacy and a fear of misunderstanding in the speaker. Misinterpretation is many times a hurdle that takes much discussion verbally to clarify. There is a tendency on the part of the speaker to leave too much unsaid or to be overwordy in this more restricted and more concrete form for the sharing of ideas.

I feel that I was especially fortunate, therefore, at the NAMT Convention in East Lansing, Michigan, to have such generous and sensitive assistance in this difficult task. Staff members of the VA Hospital at Battle Creek, Michigan, Edmund Barry, Gordon Ferris, Jay Poll, John Golden, Arthur McNeil, and Thomas Clark, acted as my interpreters, so that the audience could see and so experience the techniques of communicating through rhythmic movement.

We had all participated together in the hospital situation at Battle Creek, so that none of us were any longer strangers. This earlier experience had helped us to know one another more thoroughly than an equal length of time in some other mode of becoming acquainted.

In addition these men were able to feel with the patients whom they were representing. I had no feeling of moving with a group of people who were solely acting, but people who were expressing the emotions that lie behind exaggerated behavior patterns.

The session as presented on the stage at East Lansing was essentially the same as one on any ward of any hospital. The techniques of dance therapy, as stated in my paper, were all observable as I danced with the withdrawn or overactive patients.

Dance as an Adjunctive Therapy With Hospitalized Mental Patients

Reprinted courtesy of *Bulletin of the Menninger Clinic*, 17 (November, 1953), pp. 219-225.

It is widely held that in man's cultural development, the era of language was preceded by nonverbal communication. In contemporary word-centered societies, however, part of acculturation consists of repressing movement as a form of communication. Nevertheless, motor activity does operate unconsciously to express emotion. We unconsciously pay attention to broad, general patterns of muscular action. We expect a fearful, timid person to move with small, ineffectual movements, and a self-confident, aggressive person to use broad, directed, expansive movements.

While verbal utterance of emotion may be withheld or disguised, its nonverbal expression cannot be entirely controlled. An action as simple as walking may reflect the prevailing mood. Likewise, as a group engaged in intellectual discussion becomes emotionally involved, characteristic postural changes and movements occur, and reveal much concerning relationships within the group. When the emotion becomes powerful enough, its physical reflection cannot be ignored, whether it is expressed simply and directly, or rechannelled through the muscular rigidity of "self-control."

In the psychotic, language loses much of its effectiveness as a means of relating to others, serving as a defensive barrier rather than a means of direct communication. The seriously ill mental patient relies to a large extent on nonverbal devices for the communication of his emotions.

Since muscular activity expressing emotion is the substratum of dance, and since dance is a means of structuring and organizing such activity, it might be supposed that the dance could be a potent means of communication with and reintegration of the seriously ill mental patient. We believe we have found this to be the case.

Inasmuch as such patients also suffer from severe isolation, dance therapy serves to reintegrate the individual with the group. Although occasional sessons are held with individual patients, the ultimate aim is their participation in a group.

SETTING

In dance therapy as conducted at St. Elizabeths Hospital in Washington, D. C. and Chestnut Lodge Sanitarium in Rockville, Maryland, no restrictions are laid down as to the type of patient attending sessions, either in terms of diagnosis or in the nature or severity of symptoms. Specific patients are often referred by staff members when they believe this form of treatment is especially indicated. Otherwise, patients are incorporated into the group at their own request, through the suggestion of other patients, or by contact in ward sessions. It is our impression that an initial contact through dancing is most meaningful to the patients whose verbal communication is extremely constricted, ineffectual, threatening, or absent.

The majority of groups meet in a room set apart for dance therapy. Even suicidal and severely disturbed patients can be conducted to the dance room without mishap. Dance sessions are held on the wards primarily to establish contact with newly admitted patients.

Structuring of the Session

As they are assembling, there is a free choice of recorded music by the patients and it usually reflects their mood. To this music, the patients are free to move spontaneously either alone, with the dance therapist, or in small groups. It is the purpose of this warm-up period not only to establish the initial contacts (see under Techniques), but to drain off excitement which might interfere with an effective structuring of the session.

With a group composed largely of depressed patients, the preliminary period is relatively short, while with disturbed patients this period of exciting music, with individualistic movement, may last for half an hour.

After all or nearly all of the group have become involved in this activity, the therapist initiates, to waltz music, a circle. This particular combination of music and pattern has been found to be the only satisfactory means of involving the entire group. Following the lead of the therapist, the circle of patients goes through simple warm-up movements such as arm and leg swings, gradually moving into body stretches and body swings. By this time, some member has fallen into a peculiarly personal movement pattern, and the therapist relinquishes the leadership to this patient, encouraging the group to move with him. A succession of patients will pick up the role of leader in movement and thereafter the therapist largely plays the role of a catalyst.

The movements used in the various dance forms by the patients become broader and more spontaneous. There is also a noticeable increase in the desire and also in the ability of the group to work together in many unison patterns. Simultaneously with this movement in unison, verbal production becomes more spontaneous, body postures more relaxed, and appropriate laughter is often evoked. Miss A. verbalized this feeling by saying, "Dancing makes me aware of me and that is the only time I can be with other people." Patients who are feeling particularly secure within the group structure will give special attention to some of the group who are still withdrawn, and attempt to bring them into the circle of dance movement.

The session moves to its close with a breakdown into individual or small group movement patterns and a final period of listening to music and conversing. It is during this portion of the session that original dances are improvised. This does not mean a return to the bizarre production at the beginning of the session, when the individuals seemed isolated in their own fantasies. Instead, these dances have form and continuity and are organized in response to music rhythms being played. It is possible for the soloist to accept an audience reaction of hand clapping or a dance by the group which is similar to her own, but modified, and still return to the group when his dance is completed.

Music selections throughout the session are consonant with the prevailing emotional tone of the group. A group in which depression predominates will start with slow waltzes and progess through lively waltzes to polkas or square dance music and return to a lively waltz. With a group of excited patients, the session starts by moving to loud, lively music and ends with listening to contemplative music such as a Bach suite or a Debussy prelude.

Techniques of Dance Therapy

To illustrate some specific, detailed techniques of dance therapy, I shall describe the methods used with a group of acutely disturbed patients. The basic purpose of the therapy with these patients is to establish as direct contact with them as they are able to tolerate.

Initial Contacts: The movements used in establishing initial contact with a patient may be qualitatively similar to those of the patient (not an exact mimicking since this is often construed by the patient as mocking) or they may be expressive of an entirely different emotion with which the therapist has responded to the patient's gestures. Intense alertness is essential in judging which approach should be used so that the dance therapist may immediately establish herself as a "safe" person.

The following is an example of how the patient's muscular tensions are picked up by the therapist and carried into dance action. One patient stands hunched forward, contracted through the abdomen, his whole posture that of a person in terror. The therapist feels the tension within her own abdomen, and using this as a center of action, she develops a tension relaxation dance sequence. The original contraction she feels may be carried into an expansive movement or into some relaxed action, neither of which can be construed as threatening. In either case, it must develop from or be closely related to the patient's own contracted movement. In his response to the therapist, the patient can carry his own contraction into a similar movement, and thus help himself to break away from his fixed emotional-muscular pattern. When action with the therapist has been established, this patient may be able to move away from his fixed spot into the room. Later he may be able to dance by himself, with another patient, or, perhaps even during the same session, join the dance circle for short periods of time.

An assaultive patient, when moving forward with threatening gestures, will evoke fright in the therapist, no matter how transient. This fright usually provokes aggressive, retaliative action. If, however, the fright is put into a dance movement, such as a shrinking to the floor, and then quickly developed into a very broad, friendly, welcoming gesture, the expected retaliation is forestalled. It is vitally important that friendliness be broadly expressed in the face. If the patient continues to come toward the therapist with a threatening movement, the next resposne is usually one of steadfastness, carried out by wide, firmly planted feet and erectness of the torso, but again with no threat of retaliation. This in turn can be developed into a friendly movement, perhaps a broad reaching out of one arm or a wide, sweeping, pushing away movement of both arms simultaneously with a friendly smile.

Following this, I often suggest putting hands on each other's shoulders and pushing back and forth, setting up a swinging motion across the dance floor. This action is in essence a substitution or sublimation of the assaultive action, which for some reason had seemed necessary to the patient.

This entire sequence occurs very rapidly and is usually carried through into a strongly rhythmic dance with much foot and leg action, such as stamping or leaping, always maintaining "reaching-out" movements toward the patient. The usual response of the patient at this time is to join in with movements of a similar quality, although of his own adaptation, and his most common verbalization at this time is to the effect, "Who are you? Where did you come from?"

Another essential element of the therapist's activity in her initial approach is the anticipation of fright in the patient as a result of the inevitable threat consequent to any contact with others. The therapist therefore, retreats from the contact before the patient does, making it unnecessary for the patient to withdraw, which would reinforce his usual mode of reacting by withdrawal. However, the therapist's retreat is never complete. I leave the patient by moving about the room in continuing dance movement, returning with a warm, friendly, inviting action.

Often, with a passive schizophrenic, who is fearful of aggressive activity on his own part, and remains rooted to one place in the room for many hours, the therapist offers both hands palms upward and moves forward and backward. Most typically, the patient's response is a fixed uplift of the hands in the same position. The therapist very gently claps against the patient's hands a few times and indicates that the movement cannot be done without his help, saying that she might hurt him (a sort of role-reversal). At this, the patient responds with a mild clapping, and as he feels release, gradually accelerates and augments the movement until it is quite actively aggressive. This pattern is interrupted when it becomes violent, through retardation of the therapist's movement and some spontaneous exclamation by her. The patient responds by continuing the clapping more gently and in conventional "patty-cake" movements and seems to feel a reduction, temporarily, of his fear of contact with others.

Although contacts are being made throughout the room on a one-to-one basis between the dance therapist and an individual patient, a number of such contacts may be taking place almost simultaneously. Dance action is so rapid and so flexible that as the therapist leaves one patient momentarily to meet another, the emotion felt and expressed by her may be changed as she turns.

During this period, the therapist has the feeling of building multiple individual lines of communication, none of which may be neglected even momentarily, and all of which will gradually be developed into a group activity, away from herself except as a catalyst.

At the moment when the patient indicates that he is conscious of dancing with another person, rather than merely accepting another dancer moving in a similar fashion, his eyes will suddenly focus on the therapist and he will touch her hands, usually grasping them hard. I always respond with a simple "Hello." Patients who have danced in this fashion often say to me, "You have known me from the beginning."

Since it is inevitable at this stage that some physical contact such as joining hands will occur, this may be a good point at which to comment on touch in dance therapy. Although the therapist always indicates her willingness, availability, or readiness to enter into physical contact by brushing her hands past the patient's up-lifted hand, reaching toward a seated patient as if to raise him up, or offering to clap hands with the patient, the act of making actual physical contact is left to the patient, whose freedom to withdraw is never restricted in any way.

It is important that there should be no attempt to alter the way in which a patient wishes to dance. At one session, Miss M. was dancing a free, elated dance to a lively polka. Her patterns were at no time orthodox polka steps, but, nevertheless, her dance conformed to the rhythm and color of the music. A new assistant, not understanding the importance to Miss M. of dancing her own polka in her own way, attempted to coax Miss M. to dance conventional polka steps with her. After a few steps, Miss M. dashed across the room, ripped the phonograph record from the machine, looked at it, and deliberately smashed it. Then she sank on a bench in a posture of despair. It was only by meeting this mood with movement and encouraging her without words to dance again in her own way, conforming to her style of dancing, that she was able to come back into the dance session.

During this period of free dance, aggressive hostility is expressed symbolically. On days when the patients have been especially disturbed, this period will be full of action expressive of destruction, either of self or others, while chants from various people will almost drown out the music. Miss E. was permitted to come to the dance room, but the therapist was warned, "Are you sure you want her? She is so unexpectedly assaultive!" Miss E. danced with intensely emotional movements during this period. Her dances ranged from those which carried her rapidly through the room with movements symbolic of destruction, to utterly despairing ones on the floor, eventually moving into action which left her whole body twisted into knots. After one such dance she smiled at me and pointing to her diaphragm, said, "Dancing comes from in here, but it leaves you feeling clean." She has never shown hostility toward any member of the dance group and is able to use the group dancing for increasingly longer periods.

Group Development: The dance therapist must use her own judgment as to the moment when the first attempt to use a dance pattern initiated by herself should be attempted. It is when the room is almost totally in action, but before pandemonium arises.

This section of the dance session starts gradually when small circles composed of varying individuals are forming, separating, and reforming. Leadership passes back and forth from members of the groups to the dance therapist and her assistants. Movements begin to lose their bizarre quality, returning to it as the circle again dissolves into individuals using movements of their own.

This portion of the session also seems to be a testing period, when patients are discovering whether or not they are still free to act as they wish within the group. As the people involved separate less frequently, verbal communication begins to develop and gradually replaces the relating by movement alone. The dance action becomes more rhythmic, and a patient can stamp his feet on the ground with awareness of the contact, beginning to relax and smile as he hears the sound of the rhythm of many feet. As a patient accepts the rhythms and begins to perform simple basic folk steps, in unison with others, his movements can be led gradually into more torso-initiated action.

At that time one frequently hears around the circle, remarks of self awareness: "This is me." "I can live." "These are my hands and those are yours." Quite as many verbalizations take the form of contrast: "I never had a friend." "This I should have known when I was a child." And again, said by too many patients to be coincidental, "My mother never taught me love. How could I learn to be with others?" When these statements are made, they are spontaneous, in rhythm to the music and dance movements, and call forth no answers, unless one accepts broader, more vigorous action of the participants in the circle as an answer.

All over-active patients have very brief attention spans and short periods of tolerance of close contact with others. Consequently, although the feeling of the growth of a group activity remains throughout the session, the shift from a large group doing unison movement to small groups and individualistic solo dancing is rapid and constantly changing.

The session ends with listening to contemplative music for fifteen or twenty minutes, with the Bach Brandenburg Concerto the favorite. During this time, the patients sit or lie in reasonable close groups, but without body contact, and there is no noise from voices. Occasionally a single patient may use the music to dance some feeling of tragedy or exaltation, but this never seems to disturb the relaxed quiet of the rest of the group.

Summary

Dance therapy, in making use of the basic form of communication, offers the individual a means of relating himself to the environment or to other people when he is cut off in the majority of areas by the patterns of his illness.

His meaningful, though bizarre movements become understandable and acceptable to others as people relate themselves to him on the basis of the emotions expressed through dance action. As his feeling of isolation and his fear of a lack of understanding are reduced, he is able to put aside autistic expression to an increasing degree, and this in turn seems to enable him to enter a group and function within it in a manner that is satisfying both to the patient himself and to others in the group.

Dance therapy is first a method for initial contact and then support. It is a warming-up medium in which a patient becomes more aware of himself as an entity functioning with other entities in comparative safety.

Dancing Helps Patients Make Initial Contacts

Reprinted courtesy of *Mental Hospitals,* 5 (February, 1954), pp 4-6, now *Hospital & Community Psychiatry*

Since the beginning of history, rhythmic action with his fellows has given man an awareness of himself as an individual. More than that, he has felt himself for the moment a part of the group, with mutual understanding and warmth. Dance, man's basic form of communication, is a way for a mental patient to make initial contact with others, to get support from the group and finally a means by which the patient becomes more aware of himself as an entity functioning with others in comparative safety is it any wonder that after dancing in a group for a few minutes, a patient will spontaneously stretch both arms and say "I feel so good"?

Let a nurse, an aide or a volunteer go on a closed ward with a phonograph or play some dance music on a piano or guitar while another shows readiness to dance, and a regressed patient will suddenly start waltzing; another will join in, and another, until the whole room is in rhythm. The patients, responding to an instinct as old as man, have spontaneously started moving their own bodies in rhythm to the music. They are using the music in their own way for their own needs.

Problem of Providing "Free" Activities

One problem in the care of mental hospital patients is that of providing a day to day schedule of activity. Many factors contribute to the almost universal problem of habitually inactive and withdrawn patients. This situation exists even in private hospitals where the ratio of personnel to patients is comparatively large, and is almost an insurmountable problem in public hospitals, where the staff ratio is necessarily small.

The majority of activities require equipment which must be under careful watch by trained workers. In many wards the use of small objects or sharp tools is prohibited for the safety of the people living there. These tools must be used in shops or on wards where people are not too impulsive or unpredictable in their actions.

But on wards where the patients either have very little initiative or are restless with short spans of attention, boredom is a problem with which nurses and aides must constantly cope. Ward duties fill short periods for a few. But for many, there are days on end with almost no activity. Radio and television are passive activities during which a patient may remain absorbed in his own feelings. Card games and reading fill much time, but not days that add up to weeks or even months. Just sitting can become a habit pattern too difficult to alter even when an opportunity to do something else presents itself.

Yet talk with the ward personnel of any mental hospital, and they are eager to tell you of the enthusiasm of the patients for the social dances held in the recreation halls. They tell you that this is one activity which needs no over-urging or coercion for patient participation. It is, they add, a severe disappointment for any patient to be left off the list. Yet these dances can be held only once a week, once in two weeks or once a month. Only patients who can tolerate a large group for a fairly long time with limited supervision can be allowed to go.

Why not break the habitual ward lethargy by dancing on the ward too? Since there is this eagerness to dance, why not make use of it in a constructive way? Many hours of relaxation can be enjoyed both by patients and personnel even without the guidance of a trained leader.

Group dancing is satisfying, not only to those taking part in the dance, but also as a passive recreation. Rhythmic action when watched is felt by the onlookers in their own musculatures. Eyes lift toward the dancers, bodies noticeably relax, and smiles appear. Suddently another patient leaves her chair at the back of the room to join the circle of people stretching their bodies and then relaxing in time to the music. It is not the urging of the leader. It is the contagion of rhythmic body action which draws her into the circle. She had made a beginning toward living and the enjoyment with others of this living.

If dancing is a part of the recreation program of her hospital, she will progress from occasional ward dances to modern dance sessions in a room used only for this purpose and then to other forms of dance of her own choosing. The role which dancing plays for her may change as she becomes ready to leave the hospital. Other activities will absorb more of her time and interest, and dancing will take its place as a medium for better body control, as a creative outlet or for social contacts, just as it might in the world outside the hospital.

Dance sessions in a mental hospital seem most valuable for the acutely ill patients and for those who remain for longer periods and who are unable to make use of activities which require verbalization, competition and individual initiative. Dance is a means of relating when other means are either restricted or absent.

Laying Authority Aside

The most difficult problem for the leader, trained or untrained, in organizing dance sessions is to grant the patients complete freedom of action. Since the structure of any hospital requires many regulations for the comfort of the majority of people, it may be hard for her to accept any and all action happening in reponse to the music. But since she herself must take part actively and with personal enjoyment and satisfaction, she must lay aside authority and become a relaxed participant so that patients may freely express their basic emotions through rhythmic action.

Chaos will not result, though if a stranger entered a session during the early part, he might feel that it had. As I am moving somewhere in the room dancing alone or with one or more patients, I have often seen a nurse or attendant take several minutes to find me in spite of my attempts to signal her in a way which will not break the action. This means that the dancing does not stem totally from my leadership. Yet out of this free expression organized activity can be developed under leadership.

Acceptance of Patients' Interpretations

Working with patients in a dance session is not working in an artificial medium, but in a very real and very primitive one. A trained leader can use this natural response to music in many ways, but it can also be used to advantage by ward personnel and volunteers who have less training but who share, as do we all, the natural love of rhythm. It is an exciting and stimulating experience for a leader to share the feeling of rapport with patients who respond to music with the rhythm of their own bodies.

The acceptance of the patients' own interpretations of the music is essential to dance as therapy. If people are allowed freedom to dance as they wish, they are as spontaneous and rhythmic as young children. But with a leader who is rigid and insistent on her own patterns and style of movement, they will withdraw from contact with others just as they do in other activities. Given complete freedom of expression, they will soon form a group which can progress to composing dances together to which they all feel they have contributed from themselves and in which they find enjoyment in working together, accepting the discipline from themselves rather than from a leader's demands.

From Personal Forms to Group's Choice

One patient for instance may have dressed herself in a Hawaiian skirt with a Spanish shawl, while she twirls and stamps her feet in rhythm, apparently oblivious to everything about her except the rhythm and the materials whipping around her. Yet with no word of suggestion, she will discard her elaborate costume and be one of the first to join the circle which is forming to dance simple, rhythmic actions in unison. She has been accepted in her own forms. Now she can accept those of the group.

Or take the unpredictable patient, given to sudden physical assaults who cannot usually share activities without someone to devote exclusive attention to her. Because of the natural fear of being hurt, many people avoid close contact with her. When she hears music, she will dance spontaneously, though in her own style. She is not yet able to take part in a dance session with conventional forms of social dancing. But if no stress is placed on the way she "should" dance, she will be able to remain with the leader and other patients for the full session. During this time, she may dance alone, with a group in a circle, with the leader alone and perhaps with another patient. She may occasionally relax in a chair, watching others dance and remain relaxed for some time after the session. The leader will find it truly fun to follow this patient's lead in her buoyant, original dance patterns and will feel empathy with her response to the music. It is satisfying not only to the patient herself but to the others to be able to feel companionship with her rather than a withdrawal.

Whether she is trained or untrained, the leader must use her own judgment as to when she should attempt gently to get the patients to develop groups. It is usually when the room is almost totally in action but before pandemonium reigns. Small circles of varying individuals are formed, separate and re-form. Leadership passes back and forth from members of the groups to the leader and her assistants. As the people involved separate less frequently, verbal communication begins to develop and gradually replaces relating by movement alone.

I frequently end a group, especially of over-active patients, with fifteen or twenty minutes of contemplative music. A Bach Brandenburg Concerto is one of the favorites. The patients sit or lie in close groups without body contact and there is no noise from voices. Occasionally a single patient may use the music to dance some feeling of tragedy or exaltation, but this never seems to disturb the relaxed quiet of the rest of the group.

As one watches these patients–very sick, psychotic patients–and Miss Chace dancing, one gains the impression that through this medium the patients have at last found it possible to step out of their constricted world and, quoting one of them, "to reach outward." Their movements seem free, easy, comfortable; they undulate, flow, and appear to express in motion and rhythm what they cannot express in words or in conventional social actions. That they can do this is a tribute to the unusual qualities of Miss Chace as a Dance Therapist but it is also a reminder to us that there are few, if any, really "inaccessible" patients.

Jay L. Hoffman, M.D.
First Assistant Physician
Saint Elizabeths Hospital

Common Principles in Music Therapy

Reprinted courtesy of the National Association for Music Therapy, Inc., from *Music Therapy*, 4 (1954), pp. 87-90.

It is gratifying that music therapy is turning its attention to the study of the needs of people in this area in specific terms, but in doing so great care should be taken that arbitrary conclusions are not drawn. Since music is recognized as a social art form it, of necessary, must be an important means of nonverbal communication. As therapy it should be, therefore, in forms that can be useful and understandable to the participants in a particular group. While much study in the evaluation of music forms that are effective has already been done, these studies are often approached with rather vague structuring and with preconceived ideas on the part of those involved. It would seem essential, however, that some goals for the therapist in music be clarified, so that each person in the field does not have to work on a trial and error basis and evolve his own theories out of his particular background, setting and experience.

There are basic reasons for sharing music in whatever setting it may occur. This effect of music is as evident in a string ensemble in a concert hall as it is in an institutional setting. An individual, whether actively or passively participating in a music session, seems to respond from his own emotions. When he is in a group of people, each in his own way participating in the activity, an empathic bond seems to be established. In the world outside of the institution, people are free either to choose their own groups for sharing this form of communication or to respond to music alone. Within an institution of any sort there is often less free choice. People are usually participants in a music session as a captured audience.

Despite this often artificial and arbitrary structuring of the group a feeling of empathy seems to exist among individuals participating in a music session. Differences in personality structure which often cause friction or indifference between individuals seem to be less obvious in many music sessions. The sharing of the music seems to form a bridge between the individuals who are present.

One problem of the music therapist is to enable people to have as much of a free choice as possible within the institutional setting so that people may feel a response to the music. It is inevitable that the therapist, out of is own needs, will feel more at home with music of a particular kind. He will, therefore, have a tendency to influence the music program accordingly. In any group of individuals who share this music with him there will always be some, and often many, who will respond with him. It is equally true that in any group some or many people will not be affected emotionally by the particular music in a particular program. It is then the problem of the therapist to lead the session in such a way that the choice is as much as possible a group choice rather than his own, and so broaden the number of people involved. When there is sensitivity to the needs of a particular group at a particular time, a powerful tool for strengthening relationships within the group is available for use. The shared emotional experience helps the individuals to feel close to one another. When this feeling of being in the midst of people who "understand" occurs, the fear of isolation from others is broken for a moment. This is no different in itself from the same experience anywhere in the world. It is only a less usual experience in an institution than in many other places. It may happen with hillbilly music in the mountain regions, with the singing of hymns in a church community, or with an evening of opera or chamber music. When the music leader is sensitive to the needs of a group, this bond is even stronger within an institution than in the world outside.

The people in an institution are brought together through the particular needs of their illness or social difficulties. Within the various groups, are people with as many differences in individual tastes, desires, and backgrounds as in a group of a similar size outside of the institution where no selective choice, on a personal basis, was used. The majority of activities in this setting are geared to treating or caring for the patients' difficulties directly. Music, however, with its ability to stimulate individual emotions, reaches through the barriers of illness. Response to the music is from the needs of the individual regardless of his particular handicap. One rarely finds a person whose music interests are different during his illness than they were prior to it, even though he may feel an even stronger need for it.

However, owing to difficulties in physical or emotional areas, people have problems in relating to others. The music leader or therapist must therefore attempt to create a climate in the music sessions in which individuals who are participating may relax and respond to the music because of their own needs and not from the needs of the leader. Members of groups should be selected for participation on the basis of their interest in a particular form of music rather than on the basis of the diagnosis of an illness, either physical or emotional. Whether a person joins a hillbilly band, the institution string quartet, the church choir or the dance group depends on his needs as an individual, not on his needs in this area as a schizophrenic or a psychopathic criminal. Only in creating the climate for the session will the leader be concerned with the illness of the individuals. As a leader, one would not expect a regressed catatonic schizophrenic to relate immediately to a large group as an active participant. But with the help of the empathic bridge of the music to which he responds as a person, and to which the leader or some one other person may respond similarly, he may dare to share his experience with that other. Gradually this bridge may be widened to contain several people without too much fear and he may feel at least temporarily that he can accept and be accepted by the group. This has nothing to do with what specific form of music was used, but that whatever form it was, the patient felt a response to it. He will respond, as a rule, when ill, to the same or similar forms of music that he did when well. The therapeutic use of this response lies within the area of making use of it as means of communication when so many ways of communication are closed to him, rather than stressing technical ability as a performer.

Evaluation of music sessions in the institutional setting are badly needed. Certainly sessions that are valuable to people with one syndrome, are not necessarily even helpful for a group with other symptoms. However, in evaluating the needs of particular groups and in what ways they are being met, a great distinction should be made between understanding what is going on in the way of relationships within the group through free communication, and what may be evaluated in terms of a particular music form. It is the structure of the session and the encouragement of initiative, spontaneity and self-confidence through the use of response to music as a tool that is the key factor rather than the attempt to pin down a specific factor in the music form itself. Similar values can be found in a session of song and a session of eager listeners at a music appreciation hour with an understanding leader. Patients are people wherever they may be, and as people they respond to music. Whether in prison, in a mental hospital, or in a school for the physically handicapped, as people they will reach out when they are truly involved in a music program. This involvement will come about when an understanding and support is given to the participants as people and not as patients. The therapist is using music to strengthen the individual's self-respect through his use of a non-verbal form of communication and so enable him to relate to others. To the degree that he feels rapport with the music therapist or the group, to that degree he will be able to lay aside, at least temporarily, the behavior patterns which isolate him.

Study can be most valuably spent in observing what was going on in the group or even in a two-way relationship when this was possible for at least some patients. The common principles in the music therapy program are not only common to the various groups making use of this tool in an institutional setting, but are also common to the other disciplines.

Music therapy has its place in the total picture of rehabilitation when the patient, in spite of his difficulties, can use it through the help of the music leader, as a means of communication or emotional expression.

Report of a Group Project, St. Elizabeth's Hospital

Reprinted courtesy of the National Association for Music Therapy, Inc., from *Music Therapy*, 4 (1954), pp. 187-190.

This past year I have had an experience with group sessions for people who had already become part of a group and felt secure, to a degree, within that group. I have been startled by what has happened. Upon returning from a trip a year ago I was met with a frantic demand, all over the particular hospital building where I work, to go to a group of patients. I thought something terrible had happened. We had had one dance session. Had I been very lacking in my perception of something that had happened? It seemed necessary to see this group of people at once.

They laid in my lap the thing that they wanted to do, a musical show. They already had some parodies written. They said, "We want to do a show about a group of women living together, and the dreams which they have, which must include men." They said, "We are a group of women who are sick. We are living together in a hospital, and so we would like to do a musical show about a group of women living together in a hospital."

They were very direct about it. The first parody they showed me made me gasp because I knew they were talking about themselves. They told me they did parodies to familar songs so that they would not be involved with poor music. One parody was to the tune of "I Hear Music,"

I hear voices, and there is no one there,
I see visions hanging in the air,
I have nightmares in the midday glare,
I wonder why, I wonder why.
Schizophrenia is new to me,
I have a double personality.
The doctors say one is enough for me,
I wonder why, I wonder why.

Then the chorus showed their own feelings. It started like this:

Take the chip off your shoulder
Take your aches and pains to Dr.—
Dr.—can help you too
Long as you can sing and laugh
You can lick most anything, etc.

The other parodies were just as much about themselves. They wanted this show to depict hospital scenes which represented what they had to say, what they had to face, how they had to live because they were sick, and what the contrast would be with what they wanted life to be like.

I was a little bit floored; I have always resisted performances. I always felt that we had to do things because we were the dance department; if one of the other departments in the hospital was doing a show, the dance department could help to do some dances. I imagined, although the patients showed much enthusiasm, some of them would find the pressure of a show too much. Perhaps this was exploiting the patients by demanding something on the basis of a relationship that was established, and they would feel obligated to make me feel happy by doing a good performance. This new project of the patients would mean laying aside some work already contemplated.

The patients' project was mammoth; they had a whole evening, a real musical show, laid out. Did they really want to do it? Was this merely something they had used to take up their time while I was away? How would the medical staff feel about it? In the plan the patients did not make wry fun of themselves as an avoidance of their illnesses. Did they really want to do this?

It was a relief, after getting medical clearance when Special Services had a Christmas show to do, so we could lay aside all of this other idea. The patients were asked if they would do this Christmas show for me. They promised to do the Christmas show only if I would promise that at the end of it we would go into this other show. There was hope, it must be admitted, that this cooling off period would serve to let them forget.

The day after the Christmas costumes were laid aside, I was met by the same patient committee with others now added to it, and told, "Miss Chace, you now have an obligation." And so, I said, "Yes, if you still want to do the show I now have to fulfill my part of our bargain."

A great deal was learned during the next few months. It was found that from the middle of January until the first week in May when we gave the show that this group could work together as a group with a common purpose. They achieved great accomplishments.

At first, I was to meet with the show committee from the middle of the afternoon on, in order for me to keep up with the rest of my program, but there was not enough time to do the job in the way the patients demanded that it be done. All of the scenes, all of the dances, all details were worked out on a group basis. This took time, and so was heard, "Miss Chace, you have to give us more time." So, it was necessary to go to the administration building, tell what was happening and ask for permission to devote my time to it.

Then came the concentrated effort, and I found that the dance department was really working harder with the patients than it had at any other time. Patients had passed through the dance sessions where they had begun to be able to express themselves in movement, and they had established a relationship with me which they felt was a safe one, so that they dared to move on. They, themselves, with a group of about thirty other patients, would offer suggestions for the show, and these would either be accepted or turned down by the committee. They learned that rejection of a suggestion was not a rejection of themselves, but that probably the group would find some other thing for them to do.

It was quite interesting to see the way the patients gave each other support. We all worked hard. We involved all the rest of the departments of the hospital in the preparations for the show, and we came through with a show that was something that belonged to the patients; it had sparkle and spontaneity. In the show they talked about themselves as people with difficulties, but with a sense of humor which was appropriate.

The medical staff was enthusiastic about the show even though the patients had established the psychiatrist as a person who plays a yo-yo and wears blinders—he took off the blinders when he read his roadmap. The nurse they pictured was always someone who was giving orders. They did not bring in the rest of the departments of the hospital, but kept it to themselves, the nurses and the doctors. They came forth with much feeling about how they would like to be. It was a good show.

Becaue of the therapeutic value from this group work, a pageant is planned based on the life of Dorthea Dix. This was suggested by the administrative directors. Miss Dix established many state mental hospitals in the United States and also established St. Elizabeth's Hospital.

I have not talked about this work with patient groups before, but now I do have something to say and the work is moving on. These are wonderful group sessions where we discuss patients' problems on a safe level. When the problem reaches a personal level it can be taken to group therapy and discussed by psychotherapists. This work may seem far removed from the work of a dance therapist, but this kind of achievement was based from, and is still dependent on, the positive relationships established in the dance groups.

"Hotel Saint Elizabeth"
A Unique Experiment in Therapy

Reprinted courtesy of *Americas*, 7 (May, 1955), pp. 33-36; monthly magazine published by the General Secretariat of the Organization of American States in English, Spanish, and Portugese.

The theater audience of a thousand people was completely absorbed in the three-hour musical, breaking now and again into laughter or applause or both. Sometimes the production evoked a mixed reaction, so that the eyes of an amused onlooker might be wet with tears. For the intent of the unique production he was watching, though concealed by lighthearted fantasy, was deadly serious. The theater was in Saint Elizabeths, the federal mental hospital in Washington, D.C., and the performers were patients. They were repeating for the press and public a show they had written and produced for other patients and the staff.

Entitled *Hotel Saint Elizabeth*, the revue was a satire on life at the hospital, "Washington's finest resort." Each act consisted of two scenes, one depicting a hospital activity, the other showing the patient's "wishful thinking" version. Miss Schizophrenia, a withdrawn, newly admitted patient—in the escape episodes she became Miss Dreamer—was introduced in the prologue, while a lusty chorus sang the "Schizophrenic Song" to the tune of "Your're Just in Love":

> I hear voices and there's no one there,
> I see visions floating in the air,
> I have nightmares in the daylight glare,
> I wonder why, I wonder why.
> Schizophrenia is new to me,
> I'm a double personality,
> Doctors say one's enough for me,
> I wonder why, I wonder why.
>
> Chorus: Take that chip off your shoulder,
> Aches and pains to Doctor Bowler,
> Dr. Twombly will help you too.
> Long as you can laugh and sing,
> You can lick most anything.
> Keep your chin up, you'll pull through!

As the dance therapist at Saint Elizabeths, I was responsible for helping to produce the show, but simply as the tail to the kite, so to speak, for the entire production was the patients' idea and carried out wholly on their own initiative. It was quite a departure in therapeutic methods. But I'm getting ahead of my story.

For the most part the patients at Saint Elizabeths Hospital are emotionally ill, many of them schizophrenics. Unlike the mentally retarded, who may need care throughout their lives, these people have a good chance of being able to return to a normal existence after a period of rehabilitation. Contrary to the popular belief that mental patients are unaware of their illness, many schizophrenics not only are alert to their maladjustments but seek help in coping with them.

In the dance department all activities are organized on the basis of group decisions. Patients are accustomed to presenting ideas for individual dance sessions, parties, special performances, decoration of the dance room, and so on; if accepted by the group, they are then carried out. Still, I was totally unprepared for what happened a few months ago when I returned to the hosptial after a two-week absence. I was told that a group of women patients, all of whom were in an acute phase of their illness, wanted to see me. Their spokesman said: "We want to do a show about a group of women living together and the funny and painful things that happen to them. Since we're living together in a mental hospital, we want it to be about us in the hospital. We can dream, too, and we do. Our dreams include men, of course, so may we invite them to be in our show?" Then they showed me the "Schizophrenic Song," written by two schizophrenics, one of whom was still hearing her "voices."

The production began to take shape. Since it was essentially a musical, there were plenty of opportunities for suggestions about songs and dances. The group as a whole accepted or rejected possibilities, deciding whether a given song belonged in one act or another, whether it should be a solo or a group number. Naturally, a few storms blew up during rehearsals, and occasionally someone would threaten to leave. Mrs. X, for example, who had a talent for writing yet is never sure that what she writes is as good as she hopes it is, wrote the prologue for the show. As with all the scripts, this was reviewed by the rest of the cast. When certain portions were cut out because they were considered too obscure or too direct, Mrs. X became angry and withdrew the script, claiming that she could sell it outside the hospital. She was assured that it would continue to be her own as part of the show; it could even be copyrighted if she chose. She was adamant. "But we need your script," someone said. "How can we start the show without it?" another joined in. With that, she gave in. As the rehearsals progressed, she never missed one, despite her frequent complaints that she was being exploited. She would make out-of-town visitors wait, explaining that she was needed for *Hotel Saint Elizabeth*.

Later Mrs. X offered to dance a tango in one scene. She purposely chose as her partner a young man who was miserably shy and consequently very awkward. She worked hard with him, and her patience and pride in his growing ease were in marked contrast to her overbearing and highly critical behavior toward other people in most situations. In both these instances Mrs. X felt a sense of belonging, and, although she still finds most relationships difficult, she at least gained a temporary satisfaction. Perhaps she can continue to teach social dancing as a career, as she hopes to do, for here she has learned to feel at ease.

The show had five acts. In the prologue, Miss Schizophrenia, alone and weary, enters "Saint Lizzie's" Hotel, which offers all kinds of services, will even "cheerfully come and get you." A barker introduces her to the people there—the nurses and attendants, ever ready to tell her what to do; a psychiatrist in blinders, who continually jerks a yo-yo up and down; and the fellow patients, who are lonely too. Miss Schizophrenia finds escape in her dreams.

In the hospital dormitory, so difficult for adults because of the lack of privacy, she dreams of a luxurious boudoir, where she is waited on by a retinue of servants; then her hero dances in and sings her a tender song. The noisy cafeteria, filled with gossipy women, becomes, in the dream-world portrayal, a fancy night club, with an M.C. who defines a psychiatrist as a "nutcracker." In the hydrotherapy scene the patients donned shower caps and draped themselves in the sheets used for this form of treatment. Then they danced and sang, to the tune of "The Whiffenpoof Song":

To the cold packs down at Hydro,
To the place where our nurse dwells,
To the dear old strip routine we do so well.
Sing we fat and thin assembled,
With our panties raised on high,
And the magic of her sprinkling casts a spell.
Yes, the magic of her sprinkling
For the aches we love so well,
In the sac-ro-il-liac
And in the joints,
We will serenade our nurse
Though aches and pains all last,
Then we'll pass and be forgotten with the best.
We are poor little girls with our minds awry,
Woe, woe, woe.
We are sorry sights but still we try,
Woe, woe, woe.
Pains that are real and pains that we dream,
Pains that we cling to through all the schemes,
Nursie have mercy on such as we,
Woe, woe, woe!

But when Miss Dreamer sleeps, she is on the beach at Waikiki.

At last she graduates from the hospital, picking up her bag and taking leave of her friends at Hotel Saint Elizabeth, who sing their farewell song, "Vaya con Dios," as she goes out to meet life again.

During rehearsal I commented that the last act did not contain the fantasy of the rest of the play. There was silence for a moment, then someone burst out, "Why, Miss Chace, that's the greatest fantasy of all—to say that we will all leave." That explained the moving quality of the last song, which never failed to touch listeners.

Hotel Saint Elizabeth gave the troupers an opportunity to portray their own delusions, their wishful thinking about life, and their anger at themselves for being dependent on the hospital staff. In discussing a scene and the reason why it must be so, they gradually developed an ability not only to work on their own individual problems of adjustment, but to help each other. This eventually led them to refer to themselves as "The Gang," an experience many had missed before they arrived at the hospital.

A number of patients who generally stayed on the fringes of such activities were absorbed into this group. They might remain aloof, rarely speaking to the others; but they made a contribution and developed friendships while doing it. Miss M had come regularly to rehearsals for two or three weeks, urged to watch members of the cast from her ward. But she would sit apart, often seeming lost in her own preoccupations. From time to time the group complained that they needed someone to take down what was said during committee meetings and the spontaneous working out of scenes. One day she whispered, "You know I could take those notes—I could keep a list, too, of the costumes and props you'll need."

Here was our script girl. From then on she wrote everything down and between rehearsals organized the dozens of lists of things we required. Later, as she sat there with her black book containing the script of the play, one and then another of the cast would consult her. "Mary, what is that line?" Mary always knew. Next she dared to volunteer suggestions when some scene was stumbling a bit. Before the end of rehearsals, when a member of the cast had to be absent at a clinic or for treatment, Miss M would offer to substitute. On performance nights, she was everywhere at once, helping with a costume or handing someone a prop. She was amazingly efficient with these people, whom she had learned to accept as friends.

Miss M is still finding it difficult to work at a job on her own initiative. When she is offered a task elsewhere in the hospital, she retreats again into her illness. But she cultivates the friendships she made during the days of *Hotel Saint Elizabeth*, when she, too, found that she could belong.

Of course, the whole cast lacked confidence. Some showed it by withdrawing; others were aggressively inconsiderate. A real stickler was one of the male leads, Mr. N, a boy of eighteen who had always been a problem. Though in many ways he had made considerable progress at Saint Elizabeths, he still did not function satisfactorily with groups. He had always entered enthusiastically into performances, playing the drums for the hospital band, taking part in choral singing, and in general playing the ringleader. But always as performance time approaches, Mr. N insisted on taking over the show. His drums would drown out the rest of the orchestra, and his demand to be the center of attention would become so annoying that the pleasure of the other participants was destroyed. In the rehearsals for *Hotel Saint Elizabeth*, Mr. N reverted to type. Not content to sing one song in a scene, he and his guitar had to do all the songs. When the others in the group balked, he either played his guitar and sang his own songs louder than those being rehearsed or left in a huff, refusing to be in the show. In previous situations like this, he had simply been removed from the group. But this time, with authority vested in the cast rather than in a single individual, he modified his demands over a period of time until he came to accept their decisions; they, in turn, accepted his leadership in many scenes. Mr. N was a proud young man as he sang and danced the romantic lead on opening night, with the support of the cast and the applause of his often indifferent family. Although he had jeopardized production throughout rehearsals, the antagonism of the group had been replaced, long before they were over, by loyalty to him.

As scenes with dialogue developed, we called on a Red Cross Gray Lady who had had experience with dramatic groups. Then dialogue and dance rehearsals were separated, with constant consultation back and forth between the adjoining rooms. New ideas sprouted thick and fast; it was no longer a question of finding enough material, but of keeping it within bounds. The men wanted to include tumbling in the beach scene, so we sought out the athletic coach. New songs were suggested at every rehearsal, some parodies, some original, and we enlisted the aid of a volunteer chorus leader. The graduation scene called for military drilling. (This was logical since many patients associate conformity to society with the requirements of military discipline; they fear authority just as the cadet fears the drill sergeant, and they resent the attendant who escorts them over the grounds or to a movie or dance.) The young man who offered his services as drill sergeant revealed strong leadership ability, and his bearing improved noticeably.

The glamour of these dramatic presentations has a special appeal for the patients of a mental hospital. Apart from the acting, there is plenty of backstage work, such as making costumes, collectig properties, and painting scenery. The troupers' energy and enthusiasm infected everyone who came into contact with the show. For weeks before the performance, wherever one went in the women's wards, costumes were being made or altered. An elderly patient had asked to take over the direction of this work from the Occupational Therapy Department. Tulle skirts invaded even the nurses' stations for safe-keeping between sewing bees. In one ward old ladies strung tissue-paper Hawaiian leis, chatting happily as they worked. Somewhere else a ping-pong table had become a cutting table. In a corner a patient hemmed a scarf. Some, too restless for the fine work, tied the raffia for Hawaiian skirts; others rolled bright-colored papers into cigarette holders. The whole building became an occupational therapy shop under the guidance of Mrs. Margaret Downes, the therapist.

To indicate the shift from the reality of the hospital scenes to the fantasy of the dream sequences, the troupers wanted a picture-frame prop. So the art therapist, Mr. Prentiss Taylor, with the help of the pre-industrial shop and the patient-assistants, fashioned a cloud that when lighted seemed to float airily. Designs painted on hospital screens also depicted the satire visually.

Eventually, all the hospital departments were involved. The nursing service furnished uniforms; the orchestra was ready with music; the sound and lighting men moved in; even the firemen found ways to fireproof the home-made equipment. After three months, the show was ready to go on.

One of the phrases heard most frequently in a mental hospital is "patient-centered activity," but as a rule it might better be labeled "staff-centered." Hospital recreation staffs are inclined to take it for granted that mental patients prefer to participate in staff-planned activities because they need backing to carry out their own ideas. Therefore, generally the inspiration for a production, the time for its presentation, and the form it will take are staff decisions. Patients eager to participate are easy to find. But because they are carrying out someone else's idea, the task of holding their interest becomes a major obstacle to production. The director may well question whether the patients are really interested or whether they are simply demonstrating personal loyalty. This is bound to show up as the time for the performance draws near, when the usual stage fright of any theater group is exaggerated manyfold. That is what made *Hotel Saint Elizabeth* particularly interesting to me. Soon losing its casual attitude, the group became almost as self-critical as a professional company. In a large hospital like this there are many activities going on to relieve the tedium, and, as a rule, special projects are not allowed to encroach on the regular schedule. I had thought that occasional rehearsals would be enough; but the patients requested more and more until my entire time was given over to this project. They practiced religiously, even outside rehearsals, and at the end of the first performance, the group insisted: "Now we can make the show even better."

The goal of all psychiatric hospitals is to restore patients as rapidly as possible to a normal life. Since much of the rehabilitation (which begins when they enter the hospital) depends on ward and recreation activities, theatrical events that allow patients to demonstrate initiative, develop self-confidence, and learn to work under discipline toward an obvious goal are extremely useful. If these activities are carried on in close cooperation with the medical staff, the patients get the maximum benefit. But even when, as happens in most mental hospitals, there are not enough psychiatrists to keep track of such programs, this form of recreation is a valuable means of release and of learning group activity. Showing such productions before the general public not only helps the patients; it also improves the outsider's understanding of mental illness.

Dance Therapy for the Mentally Ill

Reprinted courtesy of *Dance Magazine*, 6 (June, 1956), pp. 36-39, 59.

Developments in "cutting through the isolation of mental patients" is a gravely serious matter to members of the medical profession, who put the welfare of their patients before any thought of casual experimentation. The author of this authoritative article on a very interesting and delicate subject was personally recommended to DANCE Magazine by Dr. Karl Menninger, as being a leading dance therapist. She is currently on the staff of St. Elizabeth's Hospital in Washington, D. C. *L. J.*

The use of rhythmic action or dance is a helpful group activity for people who are emotionally disturbed, not because of their illness, but in spite of it. Response to rhythmic sound throughout the body, not alone by ear, is a basic response. Long before a baby begins to use words, he moves his body in response to music or a rhythmic percussive sound. How many dance teachers have had the mothers of small children come to them convinced that these children will be great dancers because they danced (or really bounced, and waved their arms to music) as soon as they could move about? Many people who feel that they cannot dance, move in free rhythmic forms when they are alone and unobserved.

In our word-centered culture we find it difficult to think of any group of people who find it impossible, or only rarely possible, to use words for the purpose of communicating with other people. Yet this is the case with the majority of mental patients. This doesn't mean that they necessarily belong to the group of patients who are so emotionally upset that they are unaware of their surroundings. Anyone who is very preoccupied finds it difficult and burdensome to sustain a conversation for more than a very few minutes.

Consequently, art forms for the purpose of communication are of great importance to these people with intense problems. Through these media they may dare to express a grcat deal of feeling that they would find it impossible to talk about: painting, music or dancing offer ways to communicate with others at a time when the usual means of verbal interchange are largely cut off from them.

Music and dance have the added advantage of being social arts. One may paint in privacy, shut away from others, even though one is giving expression to inner feelings. Music and dance are more easily shared. Only if someone plays an instrument in a sound proof room is that sound not shared by another person at the time the music is being played. When the player is one of a group of people blending sounds on various instruments, he not only shares the music with a listener, but he also shares the making of that music with other peolple. Dance goes one step further. Since it involves an individual's body, he is more involved in the activity with others than through the use of music that he is making on an instrument.

I remember one young woman who had been staying away from most people for a period of several months. However, she did occasionally join with others in dancing or moving rhythmically in circular formation, where she was able to remain for long periods of time. Suddenly, one day, as the group was resting, she jumped into the middle of the room. She pulled her elbows tightly against her body and started to walk across the room saying, "All the days of my life I have been pulling in and in and in to myself. But now I can feel myself go out from myself."

There have been many ups and downs in her illness, but she has always wished to come to the dance sessions. Many times when I saw her on her ward she would tell me of other patients who should be encouraged to come with us. It was interesting that the people whom she wished to have encouraged were those who were sitting apart from others in the room. As time went on she was able to participate in group therapy and many other recreational activities, but she never scheduled other activities at the time of the dance sessions. Very early in her illness she was able to speak of the feeling in herself that dancing was able to give her, and which stayed with her in her progresss toward health.

Singing for close contact with others is similar to the use of dancing, but again falls short of involving the whole individual. When people are joining together to sing a familiar song, it is a joy to watch their faces relax and an expression of happiness with occasional smiles replace a more usual expression of sadness or anger. If, in addition, the group that is singing is also moving, speech may begin to take place between members of the group and the bodies will also relax. In many places in the world, song and movement are accepted as belonging together. When we remember that we feel rhythm in our whole body, it is more basic to move as we sing. Although we accept this point of view for small children, we sometimes forget that, as adults, we feel this same impulse to move as we sing.

Our culture demands that we move in prescribed established patterns, which are learned forms, if we wish to call these rhythmic patterns of movement dance. However, free forms of movement are often more rhythmic than our accepted forms of dance. They are spontaneous, direct and highly imaginative. The true artist retains this spontaneity and originality and, with added technical ability, achieves the statement of an idea through the acquired skill. However, in dance as in other arts, a person too often is content with technical skill, and the final result is a sterile form devoid of meaningful communication.

The extreme opposite to this stereotyped mode of dance is that of the patient who is temporarily blocked in speech. He is using movement to communicate his immediate feelings. Consequently, his dance, while technically of no school of movement, is rich in a spontaneous expression of idea or feeling. He often dances alone when he hears music, as a natural activity.

Dance therapy is making use of this natural response to music by the patient.

At the moment that a mental patient arrives in a hospital, he begins to enter into activities which the doctors feel will be helpful to his rehabilitation and return to the outside world. He is usually overly quiet or extremely active with rapid changes of mood. He also has very short spans of attention.

In hospitals where there are not enough psychiatrists for intensive therapy to be a part of every day living, helping patients to use their time constructively becomes a serious problem.

Even in a hospital where intensive work with a psychotherapist is the principal treatment, there are still many hours of the day to be spent in just living. Often, time is spent aimlessly or in a desultory fashion. People who are severely disturbed emotionally are often so pre-occupied with thoughts of their own problems that they have little energy left for concern about the place in which they are living, other people who are sharing their environment, or what is going on in the way of activity.

Any activity that requires the amount of concentration considered usual in the average group outside of he hospital, is possible for only a small number of patients. Games or sports require the element of competition. Again, only small groups can tolerate organized team play, the rigid limits of rules, and the possibility of defeat. Books furnish a retreat for a few, but not for the vast majority.

When the dance leader enters the ward where the patients who have recently entered the hospital are living, she will find the majority of people either sitting, walking about restlessly or writing at a table separate from the group. Two or three may be facing the televison, perhaps watching, although with little apparent response to what they are seeing. One or two may be playing a card game with a student nurse or possibly talking with her. There will be little feeling of group interest.

When the phonograph and records arrive with the dance leader, some people will show an interest. Someone will set up the phonograph; someone else will examine the pile of records to see if there is anything that interests them; someone else will begin to dance along as the music is heard.

The first goal of the leader in this situation is to break through the isolation of individual patients, with movement, and help them to be able to accept another person without fear, if only for a few minutes at a time. This can be done only by accepting the way in which the patient is moving and by withdrawing when the patient has has this close a contact as long as he can tolerate it for that time. She begins to move with the patient who has started to dance as the music was first heard. Perhaps the leader will be accepted; perhaps, on this first contact, she will not be. Now others will be beginning to move. Someone will accept the leader but only if she can move in the rhythm and the manner of the patient. If a dance either lacks spontaneity, or for one reason or another she must dance in her own style, nothing will happen in making a relationship. Perhaps the patient will merely ignore her, perhaps stop dancing or perhaps show intense anger.

At one session, a young student who danced well in her own style, was unable to accept a very exciting dance by a disturbed patient who was using a polka rhythm to express some intense feeling. The patient pulled away from her, rapidly ran across the room, ripped the record from the phonograph, continued her running until she was in a far corner of the room, sat looking sadly at the record, and the smashed it across her knee. Her dance had been destroyed and she found it impossible to return to the dancing at the session.

If the student had been able to adapt her dance action to that of the patient she would have begun a relationship that could have cut through the isolation at least temporarily. Often a patient who has been accepted in her own dance movements can then join a group activity in dance which is more usual in form. Often conversation will develop in the group and speech will accompany the body actions. When this happens, the group is usually moving in a circular formation with simple actions that are basic in form.

It is essential in sessions with the very isolated patients for the leader to be aware when they are expressing emotions of importance. This is equally true when people who are convalescent are working with a group on dance compositions. As in any group working on creative dance, it is vital that the leader not dominate the group with an insistence upon her own style. If the technical structure is so rigid that attention is focused totally on the learning of technical skills within a very close limit, a great deal may be achieved in this area, but with a dearth of spontaneity on the part of the students. In the hospital setting and as a part of the whole program for the patient, it is even more essential that attention be placed on the movements of the individual members of the group—and these be encouraged, especially in the hospital setting where rhythmic action is being used as a tool for patients to accept one another. Nothing will happen within the group if the leader is concerned, either totally or in a large measure, with the dance action as such, and if she dominates the group with her own style of movement. Only through constant awareness of the changes in movement by the various individuals may this be achieved.

The passing of leadership in types of movement from one patient to another is one necessary part of achieving this goal. This can be accomplished without words but by movement alone. The leader adapts her action to that of one of the patients who is doing a dance of her own. When the group follows, the new leader will show great pride in her whole posture. She is doing, for the moment, something that is acceptable to others, rather than something which she feels is unacceptable.

Another value of dance and perhaps one of the most important, is that of furnishing a tool to the patient to become aware of himself as an entity. Any dancer is conscious of an added awareness of himself as he moves freely and with his coordination as keen as possible at a given moment. Imagine how much more satisfying this can be to a person who is apt to feel his body inept, lethargic, or even unable to be moved about.

One young woman with stooped shoulders and a dragging step as she entered the dance room, began participating vaguely in the relaxing exercises of the group. Suddenly as she stretched lackadaisically upward, her whole manner changed. She suddenly began moving with energy and her face relaxed. She stated with excitement, "I can feel myself. Now I can be with the rest of you."

Another young woman was pushing in a swinging motion with the dance leader who was exerting very little energy. The patient said, "Please push harder. You feel as though you aren't there." As the dance therapist began to push with energy and accepted strong pushes from the patient, her face lighted up and she smiled as she said, "Now I can feel you. You are there and I am here." It might not seem important to know this—it is an everyday experience for most people. But to people who are uncertain about everything, nothing at that moment could be more important.

Each activity in the hospitalization of a mental patient is of help as one facet in the whole program for his recovery and rehabilitation. Rhythmic action in group situation helps him to express feelings in action patterns in an acceptable way and in an activity where he can feel that he has something to contribute at a time when this is rarely true. Dance is an adjunctive therapy. It is useful in the broad picture of a full program. No patient could be cured by dance. However, when it is important to find every possible means for helping a mental patient to be self aware, gain confidence, self respect, and initiative, to learn to accept himself and other people, dance can be a very useful tool.

The training of a dancer who is interested in using the dance with hospitalized mental patients, should help her to use this medium as a tool for helping others to feel at ease with a group, form relationships on a non-verbal level, express emotions in movement terms, and begin to feel self-respect and acceptance in living. This means that in addition to dance background and personal spontaneity, a dance therapist needs study in group leadership, knowledge of behavior patterns, and treatment methods; plus supervised clinical experience in a hospital setting. With such training, a dancer can find a satisfying and rewarding life for her love of the dance in a new field that badly needs qualified people.

Measurable and Intangible Aspects of Dance Sessions

Reprinted courtesy of the National Association for Music Therapy, Inc., from *Music Therapy*, 7 (1957), pp. 151-156.

Every person engaged in the use of the arts in a hospital situation today is constantly under pressure to participate in structured studies for the purpose of evaluating accurately and objectively what role the art sessions play in the treatment of patients. Those who are leaders in these activities are often accused of being too vague in the use of language and other symbols, so that the terms they use have little or no meaning to the other disciplines in the same environment. Since we live in an age of dependency on standard criteria for evaluation of myriads of facts, these criticisms are valid. We are dealing with the often intangible interpersonal relationships affected by shared emotional experiences. We often evaluate what is going on through our own feelings or empathy, for which, of course, there is no possible means of validation.

Perhaps in the area of painting, where the product of an individual remains visible indefinitely, some scale for the evaluation of the more gross responses and the overt changes in a participant of painting sessions can be devised and may have some validity. Too often, however, the art therapist falls into the trap of using such scales for diagnosis alone, or resorts to a shift to verbalization by the patient rather than using the art product for his evaluation and interpretation. When such evaluations are published, the reader is confused as to what was an interpretation of a verbal exchange between the patient and the art therapist and what really went on in the nonverbal area of the art communication.

A considerable amount of attention is being given to the nonverbal forms of communication, often with very little understanding of the difficulty in the translation of these happenings into verbal terms. More is lost in this translation than in the translation of word symbols from one verbal language to another. An example of this might be that of a man in one of the groups recently being studied at Saint Elizabeths Hospital who gives an outward appearance of stolid and almost sullen passivity. For six sessions this man had remained very withdrawn, although he had participated in the group rhythmic movements. During this period he had not spoken nor made either a friendly or a hostile gesture toward anyone. The group began working on strong movements which were often aggressive, in order that they might feel positive body action rather than limp half gestures. The man previously described was asked to drive out his fists in an aggressive action toward the dance therapist, who was doing the same action toward him. It was necessary for him to walk considerable distance to reach her. This he did, without hesitation, and when he was in front of her, he reached out his arms in a tender manner, (again a descriptive phrase unacceptable to standardized scales) placed his hands under her arms and stood for a moment relaxed in front of her before he returned to his place in the circle of people in the session. In spite of the refusal to respond to her request the dance theapist experienced no rejection, but rather a dependent reaching out from him combined with a comforting gesture.

Following this incident, the patient took a more positive role during the remainder of the dance session, and at the beginning of the following one was ready with a handshake and a smile as he entered the room. On any logical scale for evaluation of group interaction he would have received a plus for showing initiative in moving across the room to the leader, but a minus for refusing a given activity. There seems to be no known scale for evaluating in a positive way what apparently went on in the emotions of this man during his action with the dance leader. Nevertheless, this is the sort of response that seems to be important to patients in dance sessions and seemed to be some sort of a beginning again for this man. He used his voice during the following session and has continued to use speech at intervals ever since.

I have recently completed a study with the Psychology Department of Saint Elizabeths Hospital. The actual evaluation of changes in the patients' awareness of themselves and others has been determined by projective drawing tests which were given to each participant prior to the beginning of the series of dance sessions and again at the completion of these sessions. A control group matched for Goodenough score, age range, and other data were also given these tests, but participated in no activities. All of the patients, both in the dance sessions and in the control group, had been hospitalized with the diagnosis of schizophrenia for a period of from five to twenty years, and had been refusing any therapy or participation in any activity for a considerable period of time. We were interested in whether there would be any measurable changes in the projective drawing tests of the patients participating in the dance at the end of twenty-one sessions, and whether these changes would be greater and of a different sort than those in the drawings of the patients in the control group.

Two objective observers were used to tabulate, at five minute intervals, the degree of movement of all participants of the dance group which seemed to be related to the music or the specific activity, and a second scale to show the breadth and energy of movements made by individual patients. As a subjective observer, I attempted to evaluate the degree of participation of each patient as a member together with his initiative within the group. If accurate, this scale would show awareness of others by the individual members, and, also, their integration into the group. I used, as a base, the apparent mood of a given patient at the beginning of each session as shown by his body action. The scale was divided into five points for rating the degree of participation in the group activity and the patient's more obvious reactions to other members of the group in relation to his mood at the beginning. The results of these scales were shown on a graph for each individual patient and have been correlated with the other scales, even though they were evaluated by a subjective observer.

I have resisted submitting to a structured study for a long time, even though curious as to whether some of the factors which I believe are tangible evidence of change in some patients, may have some correlation with those things which are actually measurable in terms of the specific psychological tests in common use today. The realization was a happy one that the psychologists were as ready to acknowledge as I was that the leader of a dance session could not function as one of the objective evaluators of the dance sessions for this study. The leader must be personally involved with what is going on or there is no session in a therapeutic setting. The human relationships in this situation are the important factors both to the leader and to the patient participants. Force and frequency of movement, and to a degree, group awareness can be measured. But are they the really important things to be measured? Are any of these aspects of the dance sessions different in any way from those of any group engaged in any activity at any time?

It was found that we can measure in a satisfactory way all those factors in a dance session which are no different from sessions of any other activity. However, the things that belong specifically to the rhythmic action and the relationships established through these have no possible base for the scale in use today.

If music, or the dance, or any of the arts are of value to patients, it is because of the intangible happenings which have no base for measurement. The outward signs of what happens to a person as he listens to music that is satisfying to him, or moves to this music with an awareness tha he is doing so, can be observed in a more or less adequate way, provided the observer is alert and sensitive to the myriads of infinitesimal changes in body posture, facial expression and breadth of movement of the patients. But how does one evaluate these changes by means of a standard scale? If the face becomes relaxed and the body at ease, rather than apparently tense, does it mean that the patient is responding to the tonal sounds and rhythms of the music, or does it mean that there has been a recall of some previous happening due to the music? Even if it were possible to measure the degree of relaxation in the body of a patient, at any given moment, that in itself is not what makes hearing the music important. The emotions which are experienced within the patient are the important things. Where would one start as a base? So many variables are present in even one simple response. Is the patient particularly susceptible to harmonious tones; is he familiar with the music; has he a knowledge of instrument playing and thus identifies with the musician; is he susceptible to suggestion? These are only a few of the variables to be considered, quite aside from his relationship with the musician. When dance movement is added to the hearing of musical tones, even more areas for possible misinterpretations are added to those already mentioned, and one is in a quagmire of variables which are impossible to account for or to eliminate. Is it more valuable, both to the leader and to the individual patients, to keep a record of what went on in any given session on an observation level, or is it more important to a measure the number of times a person moved, or the force in actions that can be observed by means of established scales?

Mrs. X often moves passively through a dance session, accepting the movements initiated by the leader, or other members of the group. Often, however, during the session, she smiles to herself and then her movements have a quality of originality and sensitivity. They are too varied to be followed by anyone else, and they will occasionally lead her to dance away from the group with an appearance of enjoyment, but with no apparent awareness of the group activity. After so doing, Mrs. X will sit by herself for a few minutes and then return to the group activity. These periods of sitting by herself decreased materially during the course of the project. The first session she sat alone the full hour with her back to the activity, but during the latter part of the series of sessions the majority of her time was spent with the group, and she left the activity only at infrequent intervals.

Which tells more about the enjoyment she is experiencing in music and movement—the description of her behavior, or the graph made from the standard scales showing her progress from isolation to partial participation in the group? How do you meansure the satisfaction she is experiencing as she does her own movements alone and apparently unaware of the group? Her movements were not large and energetic; she left the group, and she frequently sat quietly when activity was being tabulated. Consequently on each scale she would be evaluated in the lower level of participation. Yet, as the leader of the dance sessions, I feel that she enjoyed the sessions as much as, and perhaps more than any of the other members. There are no statistics to confirm this—rather the reverse, but when consideration is given as to what dance means to people on an emotional level, the leader can sympathize with her and recognize that she has had an enjoyable experience at each session.

An extreme example of another patient who gained little if anything from the sessions as measured by our scales was Miss Y, who remained almost totally quiet throughout the twenty-one sessions, although she stayed in the group formation. The majority of the time she did not even participate in movements which were being done around her. But at intervals, when especially selected, she attempted to lead an activity even though she used very small and inadequate movements. When she was able to do this her face became radiant and alive. Again, on the scales she is almost at the bottom of the list. But who can say what those rhythmic actions mean to her when she is able to move, however inadequately. How can you rate a smile; how can you rate the reaching out of hands to a trusted person for a few minutes at a time?

It is right that attempts should be made to evaluate benefits to patients from participation in music and dance sessions. If it were not that such participation is beneficial in some way, these programs would have no place in a hospital setting. The question is whether the descriptive method is not really more adequate for true evaluation than the present day "so-called" scientific scales of measurement. Not only do they show only the most obvious changes and happenings, but also, they are tabulated by people. This of itself brings in a subjective viewpoint, however objective the observers may try to be. Are these evaluations really more scientific than the observations of the person who is responding to a patient's movements on a feeling level?

While we are involved in listening to music, or playing it, or using our bodies in response to it, we are involved in a feeling experience. If this is so difficult to translate into verbal terms in any way, how can one hope to translate this experience into meaningful symbols for the purpose of statistical information? It is easy to know how many people participated in a session, for how long, and with how much increase in motor activity. It can be known whether these facts coincide with possible changes in a projective drawing test. But what then? Does this tell anything of the shared experience of the group members, the enjoyment, the growth of awareness of the music, or the friendships begun and their meaning?

Are we, as artists and musicians, lending ourselves to projects for evaluation which tell less of the true meaning of these sessions to the patient than the ones we are now using? It is true that the DAP tests in this specific project showed phenomenal change for the majority of patients in the dance sessions. Although all thirty-five patients, both men and women, had been hospitalized for periods of time ranging from five to twenty years, only five did not show a change of one to twenty-one points in the two tests. One of these refused to attend, and two others were able to come only occasionally. On the contrary, the members of the control group either showed no change or showed less awareness of the body image on the second test, again with the exception of two who improved. However, this has been obvious from the total picture of improvement without the tests and without the laborious mechanisms involved in tabulating the objective observations. They indicate no more than small facets of the total picture of social improvement.

Until there are ways of measuring the so-called intangibles, which are so very tangible if one does not require a base for measurement, perhaps it would be wiser to continue making evaluations on a clinical evel. These thoughts are not offered as conclusions, but rather as questions arising from personal experience.

Development of Group Interaction through Dance

Reprinted courtesy of Grune and Stratton, Inc. from *Progress in Psychotherapy–Technique of Psychiatry*. Vol. 3. Edited by J. H. Masserman and J. L. Moreno. New York: Grune and Stratton, Inc., 1958, pp. 149-153.

"The theatre audience of a thousand people was completely absorbed in the three-hour musical, breaking now and again into laughter or applause or both. Sometimes the production evoked a mixed reaction, so that the eyes of an amused onlooker might be wet with tears. For the intent of the unique production he was watching, though concealed by highlighted fantasy, was deadly serious. The theater was in Saint Elizabeths, the Federal mental hospital in Washington, D. C., and the performers were patients. they were repeating for the press and the public a show they had written and produced for other patients and the staff."

This is the opening paragraph of an article about the first revue performed by the members of the dance group at Saint Elizabeths Hospital. But it is equally applicable to the several products which have followed this one. The theme is always one concerning itself with their illness, satirical comment on hospitalization and psychiatry, coupled with dreams of a world which is warm and welcoming and where they can feel at home. In each of their productions the patients portray their own delusions, their wishful thinking about life, and their anger at themselves for being dependent on the hospital staff.

It might seem strange that elaborate products combining dance action, speech, costuming and stage properties should develop in the atmosphere of the almost nonverbalizing dance sessions, if it were not that these musical plays are largely dance dramas with a few words spoken now and then, where words are essential to the action. Although our dramatic productions take shape now at almost regular intervals, the idea for a new one develops within the group itself without any urging from staff members. One hears—either in nostalgic tones or impatient ones—the question, "Why haven't we started a new show? The last one was such fun." After an interval long enough to be sure that people are ready for working together closely for a period of time the dance leader calls a meeting of those who have been asking these questions. From then on the director feels rather like a tail to a kite. Ideas spout forth and the director's function is largely that of making sure that one person does not take over and use the group for his own self-glorification, but rather that the production moves according to a consensus of the group's wishes.

Although these productions have gained a reputation of being good theater, and consequently worth attending by the general public, the great value to the patients lies in the building of the production. For many of the people involved it is one of the rare times that they have felt a part of a group working toward a common goal. Today, the accent in a patient's daily life is placed upon helping him to function again in a community together with an awareness of himself as a person able to contribute to this community in acceptable ways. Although threater seems to some people apart from daily living, the production of a creative drama in a hospital setting furnishes a very realistic community for patients to test their abilities in these two areas.

Miss X. is a very quiet person. As a rule she stays on the fringe of a group activity. She may dance a little in a dance session when the activity is not too strenuous, but she never has the courage to improvise on her own. She seems to feel that she has little that is worthy of attention from anyone else. However, as the group discussion becomes lively and someone suggests that ideas are coming so fast that we may lose sight of some of them, Miss X. suggests to the leader in a whisper that she can take shorthand, and she moves into the group as the secretary. The name Miss X. has been used purposely as there is always a Miss X. in each production. She often leaves the role of secretary for that of an actor in one of the scenes. When this happens, Miss X. is the one chosen for the part by the rest of the group because of the sensitivity with which she has played some scene during improvisations for the show. The joy in the face of each new Miss X. as she realizes that others like her and what she does, and she is able to say "Why yes, I could do that, if you want me to," is exciting to see.

There is one tremendous difference between theater as an art form in the world outside of the mental hosptial and within it. The former is objective, and plays are developed through a knowledge of theater techniques, while the latter is entirely on a subjective level both in writing and in performing. The patients live their roles. This would be bad theater anywere else in the world except in the spontaneous dramas of very young children. The patients are also able to achieve the same quality of feeling that the children do with this method, although on an adult level. Tears are often mixed with laughter at their very real humor, and serious ideas that might have been sentimental are stark in their sincere reality. These are the aspects of a production within the hospital which makes it a living community rather than something removed from life.

The group discussions during the planning period of a production are perhaps one of the most important parts of theater productions for the patients. Since they are working subjectively in their planning, they always use their own feelings and their own experiences as gauges of the accuracy of roles in the play, of emotions to be aroused in the audience, of variety of action for sustained interest and of the forward movement of the drama. During this period when they are testing the acceptance of their feelings and ideas it seems a helpful thing to the members of the group that the emotions which they individually feel can be understood and shared by the others. Friendships develop, and warmth toward one another pervades the group in spite of disagreements and occasional hurts which can be worked through in action because of the warmth and understanding. Perhaps for the first time someone will feel a sense of self-respect in relation to other people as well as a feeling of belonging. Often at the final performance of a production one hears repeated many times, "I can give up the show, but I can't give up the gang."

The group discusses an idea for some time before they start to work out the dance patterns or the dramatic action. Many people present ideas which will be accepted, rejected, or modified by the others before the final decision is reached as to the form which will be used to present a particular idea. The members of the group accept the decisions of the group as a whole and then seem able to be wholly involved in the project. Individual members seem to hold no apparent resentment because their own ideas are not being used, If, however, at any time the leader tries to modify these ideas because of her own fear of failure, or because a theme might prove too "corny" and sentimental for her own taste, defeat to the idea will result. Occasionally an idea that seems corny or overly-sentimental in the discussion stage will prove to be very moving in its final presentation, because of the intense feeling of sincerity about it among the group members.

It is important for the leader of such a theater group to be alert to two dangers that are ever present. One is the tendency to distrust ideas that do not coincide with his own, and the other to fear that plans cannot be carried through by people who have often failed in this area.

During our production "Cry of Humanity," the group wished to compose a ballet to show the conflict exprienced by Dorothea Lynde Dix in trying to make her decision to better conditions for mental patients. Her goals were very grandiose ones, since she wished to influence the legislators of Massachusetts to build state hospitals for mental patients rather than to farm them out with private families as was their policy. She was a physically weak young school teacher who was so shy and awkward that she found it difficult to attend social functions in the Boston of the middle of the nineteenth century. Her biographies mention only that she was weary from many wakeful nights at the time she was making this painful decision. The group of patients who were doing research and composing the drama believed that thoughts of the suffering mental patients must have come to her at this period almost as intensely as their own hallucinations. They felt that they must dance these feelings as the only way to communicate them to an audience.

The leader's experience had been that as patients were again able to use speech to communicate with other people their improvisations in dance became less emotional and often were quite stereotyped. She was afraid that they would meet with failure in projecting their idea in dance form. It was foolish to have feared this; if they had been prevented from carrying out their idea in dance form because of the director's hesitancy, one of the most moving theater dances I have ever seen would have been lost.

The group chose music which would help them to feel again, not merely to recall intellectually, the emotions that they had experienced as they danced while they were very psychotic. They were able to verbalize in discussion about this, and for the first time I learned that they were aware that they had expressed fear, hate, aloneness, and all the feelings I had seen them dance. I also learned that this was not out of their awareness as they danced, but rather that they had used the dance at that time as a means for communicating these feelings.

Later the leader was able to trust the group when they planned to dance the feeling experienced in looking at a Rorschach card and the following year, a dance of death and destruction to represent the feelings of the Hungarian people in the last tragic fight for their freedom, as well as many delightful and satirical pantomimes. For such dances the group has always chosen music which was pertinent to the mood and moving to the audience. Group discussion was used in making these choices. For the mood of the Rorschach card they chose excerpts from *Jeremiah* by Leonard Bernstein; for the dance of "Death and Destruction," the *Death and Transfiguration* of Richard Strauss, and other music equally suitable.

Naturally, the people who are the performers gain the greatest benefit from these productions because of their shared experiences in the dramatic and dance action, but benefit from such an activity in a hospital setting is also gained by the people on the fringes of the production. Some older women feel a part of the younger members' activity as they sit and sew costumes during rehearsal hours. They are again active and useful members of a community which is working toward a demanding—but a not too demanding—goal. People who have made the costumes, worked on the staging or the theater props and who have acted as stage hands or dressers for the performers know that the show could not have happened except for them. They share in the applause of an appreciative audience.

Patients are often unaware of or take for granted the care which the personnel whom they rarely see give them. The dietitian is rarely thought of as a person. She suddenly comes alive when she prepares a picnic lunch for an all-day rehearsal at the theater. The carpenters who occasionally pass through a ward or a corridor with a box of tools are ordinarily people far removed from the patients. But when the carpenters make a piece of scenery from a patient's design, they suddenly become aware of the contributions of the carpenters to their care, not only in relation to the show but in their day to day living. Through a theater production patients can become part of a hospital-wide community that cares about what happens to everyone.

Theater productions by patients are not only fun mixed with hard work which have glamor and applause as a reward, but they are also one way of structuring a kind of living that can be shared with others and in which each patient and member of the personnel involved in it can give of himself to a common goal. For a time, the patients can experience while they are still within the hospital some of the healthy aspects of living in a community outside the hospital.

Stimulation of Creative Forms in Patient Productions

Reprinted courtesy of the National Association for Music Therapy, Inc., from the *Bulletin of the National Association for Music Therapy*, 7 (September, 1958), pp. 9-10.

(*Summary of a paper presented at the Fifth Annual Southeastern Regional Conference, March 7-8, 1958, South Carolina State Hospital, Columbia, South Carolina*)

The use of the term "creative" in conjunction with any of the arts is a must for the description of classes today. Whenever one picks up a periodical which advertises classes, one sees the use of this term—creative drama, creative art, creative dance. Often in visiting such classes one seeks the justifiction for the use of this term in bewilderment. What is meant by the teacher when he uses it? Only occasionally one finds a truly creative session and then it is an exciting experience. Usually, it means a rigid conformity to the ideas of the teacher. How sad that an expression so meaningful has become such a sterile cliché.

I believe that dance (which to me is the most vital and the most personal of the arts) is perhaps the worst offender. Because it uses the body of a person as the tool for communication, dance becomes a direct communication from that person. Instruction is given for the most part through observation of the teacher's movements. Inevitably there will be a tendency on the part of the pupil to mimic as exactly as possible the movements of the teacher. Here arises one the major difficulties in making dance classes a truly creative experience for the pupils. There is a natural admiration of the pupil for the teacher and therefore, a preconceived idea that her movements should be emulated to be correct. The strong narcissistic feeling on the part of the teacher, and the fact that her style of movement is the most satisfactory way for her to move, combined, quite practically, with the need to demonstrate ways of moving that will give the most efficient use of the muscles, cause many blocks to true creativity for the pupil. Often, the teacher is so flattered by seeing duplicates of herself moving about that she forgets that no two people have exactly the same body nor exactly the same feeling about the use of that body.

Not all people are artists but all people can be creative. The artist dancer has the ability to absorb feelings and ideas from the environment, and through a point of view belonging peculiarly to himself, give back to others his comment on these feelings in a way that is understandable to those who participate as an audience in his communication. Only rarely does a teacher have the opportunity to nurture the development of the artist dancer. One can never teach the artist dancer in the most strict sense. He already knows what he must say before he begins to develop a technical equipment with which to say it. One can only help him to develop the skill which will enable him to speak in more and more eloquent terms. These are not the kind of people one finds in the usual student dance group. Rather, one finds people who have things to say but are often blocked in the saying; those who can find great joy in the expression of feelings and ideas although they are not driven to speak the intensities of these feelings. These are the people who can more easily conform than not conform; who rarely have anything to say which has any importance for others to hear. They do have their own way of thinking and of moving. This belongs to them and seeks expression.

The teacher or leader, depending upon the situation, is obligated to support the tentative expressions of personal feeling of the members of the group. These are often shown by the individualistic ways in which a basic technical movement is approached. Certainly it is important to have as much knowledge as possible of proper ways of moving and accepted technical forms of dance action in order to be as free as possible in the use of the body. A class centered around simple forms of efficient ways of moving can both begin to develop a vocabulary and also teach the pupils that their way of doing the movements is worthwhile.

Perhaps one develops a respect for the ideas of others through the tireless and patient efforts of his own teachers. In whatever way it develops, this must be the attitude of the leader of a group if, in turn, the group is to have respect for the efforts of individual members. This is necessary whether the group is in or out of a hospital situation. In some ways the development of this climate for a creative group is more easily achieved within the hospital, and in some ways it is more difficult.

One asset in a group of psychotic patients lies in the fact that they are so absorbed in their own thoughts and feelings that it is difficult for them to accept other ways of thinking and feeling. In this they are similar to, but not the same as, the artist. More original ideas will come from a group of mental patrients when they are in a climate conducive to the expression of ideas than will come from a community group of similar size. People learn at an early age to conform to accepted ideas.

In the hospital dance sessions all ways of moving are accepted. Rhythms that are unusual, but have a direct relationship to the music, also are accepted. These are direct expressions of the people involved and as such deserve respect. This develops a climate which the patients refer to as "peaceful." I am often startled by the use of this term as it may have been said on a day when there was a great deal of activity in a comparatively small space. However, for the participants, it was peaceful.

It is in this climate that ideas are developed for patient productions at St. Elizabeth's Hospital. I am always startled by the suggestions as they never are things I could have planned. Since individuals' movements, expressions of feeling, and behavior patterns have been accepted, it is easy for them to expect that others in the group will be willing to help carry out an idea. When a patient develops this belief, he has become a part of the group.

In planning for the holiday performance last year, it was suggested that we might do scenes from the life of Christ rather than scenes stopping with the nativity. The group decided that Jesus the baby was important because of Jesus the man. I had been content to leave Christmas with the babe in the manger. The idea of the group made me stop and look again at my own concepts of Christmas. In the last scene, a ballet in which human moods are the reason given for the conquering by devils, I was startled by the choice of moods—not the ones considered as wicked and evil, but, rather those of weakness, depression, vanity, jealousy, and cowardice. My choices would have been rage, hatred, avarice, and all the intense destructive emotions. Perhaps the patients were right. The devils' costumes did not look like devils. They were gay with only stylized horns and tails. The reason? If one knew that a devil was a devil, one would avoid him and not submit to him. How true, although few people would think of devils from this point of view.

If my own concepts had been used as the format for our holiday show, it would have centered as usual around the birth of the child Jesus in one way or another. By listening with close attention to ideas from the group of patients, we had the basis not only for a new theme, but one which had a point of view which could stimulate new thinking.

One of the difficulties in working with a group of psychotic patients seems to be that their point of view is often difficult to understand because of a lack of relationship to the total picture. However, if the production is to be theirs and not the leader's, it must be built from their concepts. The bridge to understanding by the audience is the major task of the leader. This is done, not by modifying the ideas arbitrarily, but through group discussions of the patients involved.

Another of the difficulties found in developing productions in a hospital setting is that of helping patients to sustain an interest in the completed play or concert. I am frequently startled at the similarity between a performance by mental patients and a marionette show. One can almost see the manipulation of the director whether he is actually in view or not. The attention of some patients wanders and they frequently become lost in their own preoccupations until someone arouses them and they become aware of what they are doing. Obviously this is not a creative patient production when this happens, and I often wonder what satisfaction was derived from the experience by the patients. Certainly, the director probably derived a certain gratification from seeing something that had required many painful rehearsals performed in a fairly adequate way with only a few upsetting incidents. What went on, however, that had to do with a better feeling and pride in a group activity is difficult to visualize. One even wonders if the experience was a therapeutic one.

The essential responsibility of the leader of a production group is to enable patients to become involved in the production as a living experience. This can be done only by organizing the activity so that patients wish to contribute to it and feel that it is their own production to which they are giving their time and energy. It is amazing how much responsibility individual patients can assume, not only for themselves but for the rest of the group, if they are given the opportunity. In carrying out a task to completion, they have taken a position of esteem and prestige in a community once again, even though this community is a temporary one and comparatively short lived. It is, however, not an unrealistic one and is frequently a stepping stone to responsibilities in a larger community. Some patients take the responsibility of costume making, others may work on scripts or programs, and still others may make props or scenery. Whatever they do, they must be permitted to work out the problems involved in their own way and at their own way and at their own speed.

Again, this is the responsibility of the leader. Many people who have rarely carried out a project from an initial idea to a completed task can do so when pressures are reduced. One of the most frustrating pressures is that of fear of failure. Too frequently this prevents many patients from participating and only frustrates their own initiative. Perhaps faith on the part of the leader is one of the important qualities in the reduction of pressures on the patients—faith that an idea is useful, faith that it will be carried through, and faith that it will be a worthwhile final product.

Dance in Growth or Treatment Settings

Reprinted courtesy of the National Association for Music Therapy, Inc., from *Music Therapy*, 8 (1958), pp. 119-122.

While there are many similarities between the use of dance in the education of the child and its use with psychotic patients, there are also many dissimilarities. Children reach out for knowledge, and in teaching them one has a feeling that all of one's resources are called upon to feed this growth. Each dance session brings new awareness of body coordination, sensitivity to musical tones and rhythms, and alertness to new ways of using the body in dance patterns. All of this is on a conscious level. The world is a curious place to the child, and he wants to find out about it.

Children have always fascinated me in their ability to absorb and retain at a rapid pace. I do not know how many teachers feel as I do, but it always seemed essential to teach them with extreme accuracy and clarity because of their ability to quickly absorb and retain the learning material.

Children are in the period of transition from nonverbal communication to communication utilizing verbal symbols. They have not yet given up the use of their bodies in direct action in response to emotion. Consequently, when they dance they often are more spontaneous and more exciting to the observer than are older peoplle, who can move with greater technical proficiency.

Most adults do not consciously employ body action as a means of communication. Consequently, they are far less alert to the meaning of movements of themselves and others. Because movement probably has less meaning to them, adults are slower in the learning process. One expects an adult group to retain no more than a third of the material given in a specific class. It is therefore possible for the teacher to make mistakes in instruction and correct the error in the following class. If this happens in a children's class one hears from all sides, "but you said." I always felt that children's classes demanded the optimum in perfection to meet this quality of alertness in the absorption of knowledge.

The teaching process is one of reeducation in the clinical situation. While it is true that during a session one has the feeling of growth, that growth is measured in small degrees of progress. Contact is made through the nonverbal communication of body action, but the patients do little reaching to the world around them. They are similar to children in their use of movement to express immediate emotion, but their movements are an expression of their inner selves rather than a response to the world around them.

The body is involved in all emotional experiences, and psychomotor tensions reveal both feelings of security and insecurity. Naturally, if one is working with children who feel a lack of trust and security in their environment, one is dealing with a clinical situation just as one is with adult psychotic patients.

As the child attains better coordination, posture, and rhythm in his movements, he often develops a feeling of greater security and confidence in himself. Many children, who are lacking in the ability to function with other children without fear, are helped materially through participation in dance classes. Grace and poise are really other names for efficient, coordinated movement and awareness of self.

With both children and mental patients it is important to remember that the dance sessions which one is leading are for the purpose of building sufficient awareness of self through expressive movement. In sessions with either group one is working for creative expression and a feeling of well being, as well as improved coordinated body action. In neither group is one working to develop a professional performer. At intervals one will find, in either group, a "poet" who is able to express ideas for others in a way that demands a specific approach in order to develop his talent. In general, however, one is working for an experience in dance that will make members of the class more confident of functioning in the world of reality rather than in the world of imagination.

It is also disastrous to use authoritarian methods of teaching in both of these groups. In a class of children one would develop a group of robots, all of whom would be weak imitations of the rigid instructor. No matter how beautiful the movements of the individual child might be, they would be meaningless as an expression of his feelings. The child performers would be technically proficient dancers with the vitality of marionettes. No contribution toward their development individual as would have been made. In conducting such a class with mental patients, one would have the patients going through movements in the characteristic dull manner of the schizophrenic. In neither instance would there be growth or regrowth.

Both groups, however, need structured classes. Each is composed of people who are dependent on authority figures and who are afraid of showing independence of action opposed to authority for fear the world will tumble in on top of them. Both groups need to be weaned from this dependency. However, both would be lost and bewildered without structure to the dance sessions. There is a world of space between rigid authoritarian domination and laissez faire. Both groups need well defined limits of expected behavior and organized instruction in the use of the body. Horizons cannot be broadened nor can the ability to walk upright toward those far off hills be developed without both limits and structure.

I speak frequently of the development of the ability to express creative and spontaneous movement in the nonverbal medium of dance. I feel that I am frequently misinterpreted as recommending free movement exclusively. Nothing could be less true. No one can speak and be understood unless he has a language which can be heard and interpreted by others.

The greatest difference in the structure of the classes for the growth of children in the educational process and the reeducation of mental patients, lies in the leadership of the two groups.

The leader is first a teacher giving instruction to the best of her ability in the children's classes. Limits are very clearly defined no matter how much initiative and independence of action is encouraged. These limits vary greatly with the chronological age of the child. Great simplicity in the structure is needed with little variation from class to class for the young child. He feels secure with known factors. There is so little he has learned and there is so much that is bewildering. As he develops he can be encourged to assume more responsibility for his actions as the limits established by the leader broaden and give him greater freedom. Even though these limits are nonverbalized and not at all times apparent, the child feels more secure in a situation where he knows they exist and where he must abide by them. The child will constantly test these limits, be rebellious at times, but will accept them and be lost without them. The child in seeking independence seems constantly to need to be sure that the leader is able to say "No" as well as "Yes."

While it is also important that the leader in a dance session with mental patients be able to set limits and, in so doing, occasionally say "No," it is far more important that he be able to set these limits so wide that they are visible only when a need arises. The person who has intense emotional problems is more frequently overdependent than overassertive. He will constantly ask that he be made to feel secure in a safe, restricted shelter. This may be done in many ways: sometimes with behavior that demands curtailment of his activity; sometimes with overpassivity that asks for constant attention from the leader; or sometimes by withdrawal from the group. The leader needs to try to help the patient to become aware of sufficient warmth and interest in order for him to dare to undertake his rightful independence and assume the responsibilities which he can fulfill.

Although the roads travel in almost opposite directions, in both education and reeducation the leader is attempting to use dance action as a means of building confidence. Both need support from the leader; both need encouragement and limits. In education the limits must be firm with a gradual widening as growth takes place, while in reeducation there must be constant alertness by the leader to attempts on the part of the patient to shrink these limits to the point where he can remain totally dependent and avoid any reaching out to the rest of the world. In other words, for the child the leader must hold firm limits which are slowly widened as the child develops naturally, whereas for the mental patient, the leader must both define limits and help the patient to push outward his own self-imposed narrow restrictions.

The Role of the Psychiatric Nurse in Dance Sessions

Reprinted courtesy of New York State Nurses Association from *SNANYS Newsletter*, 8 (October, 1960), pp. 8-9.

The psychiatric nurse is of great importance in any activity program in the mental hospital. her attitude can either augment or stultify the program of any recreation worker. This, of course, includes dance sessions whether on the ward or in specific areas assigned to these activities. Her own personality and her concept of the role of the psychiatric nurse will dictate the degee of her involvement in the programs, but this is beside the point in considering her importance in any situation involving participation of the patients under her care.

In many institutions nurses are at premium, and responsibilities of having a harmonious ward situation absorb her full attention throughout the day, the hours of which are never enough. The pressures of too much to do with too little help sometimes cause her to feel that any activity outside of her own routine duties is something that should be the total responsibility of the leader of such an activity, particularly one such as dance and exercise. This is both understandable and highly frustrating to the leader as well as the participants in the patient activity.

I sometimes wonder if the nurse in charge of a ward or the supervising nurse in charge of a building realizes the importance of her approval to the patients in her care. So much of her attention is that perhaps she does not seen herself as someone whom the patients respect as knowing what is worthwhile and helpful in a human way.

One of the major problems in any ward situation is that of motivating to activity patients who often let days and weeks go by with little or no seeming interest in people or the general activity around them. It is often such a tiring task to involve them in the ward program that it is the line of least resistance, after weeks of effort, to let them remain sitting. It is true that these patients often lack the necessary energy to participate with others in activities that require alertness, conversational interchange, skill in games or intellectual give and take, and no amount of urging would enable them to do so. Dance sessions are often able to cut through this extreme withdrawal. How wise, then, for the nurse in charge of the ward to assist the leader with her encouragement to the patients to join the group. This will more than compensate her for the time away from her other pressing duties on the ward as she will have a more cheerful group of patients, at least for a period of time.

At Saint Elizabeths Hospital it is not unusual for the nurse in charge of a ward to participate in a dance session when she has time available. If she is unable to do this she will encourage her nursing assistants or the affiliating student nurses to take an active part in the sessions. Although the question is sometimes raised to whether in functioning on a level with a patient in a rhythmic movement session her needed role of authority is affected, this never seems to be a problem where a nurse is secure in her role. Only where a person is dependent upon her uniform for sustaining her role could this ever cause misunderstanding to patients.

Dance sessions at Saint Elizabeths Hospital are conducted largely as sessions to encourage full body action by patients. Much of a session is devoted to helping a patient to use the large muscles rather than the small muscles in wrists, ankles, hands and feet. By doing rhythmic stretching and relaxing movements to music, a patient begins to move in a more complete way. This in turn tends to give him a feeling of well being and an awareness of the others with whom he is moving. Out of this develops a form of communication and understanding.

Since good psychiatric nursing of today stresses guiding the patient into areas of group interaction, broadening the patient's contacts in his environment, development of as much independence of action as possible, and similar attempts at motivating patients toward resocialization there is nothing as a participant in dance sessions (where the focus is on communication) that is outside of the role of the psychiatric nurse. It would seem to be useful to use a tool that fosters both communication and understanding.

One nurse in charge of a rehabilitation ward of men who had been out of contact with the social life of the hospital for a long time felt that ballroom dance sessions were among the greatest needs for these men. She spearheaded the organizing of such a program, making arrangements with the dance therapist and volunteers to carry on the program. Although she attended sessions only at intervals many discussions of the dance sessions took place in her group meetings and she was always felt as a part of the program.

On the other hand, although a nurse is present on the ward during dance sessions, if she feels that involvement in dance sessions is not within her role and remains in the nursing office throughout the period of time, her lack of presence is also felt. Only because the patients reach out for this form of activity can the dance leader stimulate any kind of enthusiasm, as the nurse is giving tacit disapproval. She has missed more than the patients would, however, as she has closed a door to nonverbal communication which would help her to know her patients better and consequently have less need to maintain a rigid authoritarian atmosphere on her ward.

In large hospitals where many patients are so lethargic that it is frustrating to the ward personnel to keep them active, lack of interest often develops in the personnel. We all need rewards and tangible evidence of our efforts. In this sort of situation sessions of rhythmic body action can give the ward personnel a boost in morale. Benefit can be received by them as well as by the patients. Here the psychiatric nurse can spearhead a group project with a feeling that she is fulfilling her role effectively rather than stepping outside of it.

Two graduate nurses in their field work experience were assigned to a ward which housed patients who had been in the hospital for a considerable time. The nurses tried a number of activities with a result of having only scattered participation. Since they were working on a project of group interaction they felt as though they were not reaching the goals they wished. After setting up and leading a few dance sessions they felt more at ease with their patients and could go on to other activities.

At the present time, too, attention is focused a great deal on activities that stimulate initiative. The role of the psychiatric nurse is one that presupposes attempts at understanding and communication. Often by entering into an activity that leads to more initiative for the patient, she can feel that communication between the little verbalizing patient and herself has occurred. A smile exchanged at this time may lead to a better understanding between them, and even though the exchange has been on a nonverbal level, there will be the awareness that two people have met for a moment.

This nonverbal exchange must occur many times a day during an eight hour shift, but when the participants in the exchange are moving in rhythm with others in the room, a sense of rapport is vastly increased. The shared experience of listening to music while moving rhythmically gives a feeling of well being that is a relief in the midst of many defeats.

In many instances where there is a program for student nurses

acculturation in education if the child is to live in our present social environment with any sense of acceptance by the majority of people.

The ideal of courteous behavior and the accepted standard for evaluating a "cultured, well brought up person" in this country, is one who speaks words with little change of facial expression and with as little use of gesture as possible. Even the flamboyant orator in the pulpit or on the political stump is no longer acceptable to his audience, and his listeners withdraw from such a melodramatic display. We listen today to the speaker who can present ideas in a cool, dispassionate intellectual form.

The child must learn rapidly to make the transition from his natural mode of expressing feeling to that of the adult world about him. Many times in the process he becomes overly static in his actions and often becomes very fearful of the results of any display of emotion, no matter how natural this may be. Perhaps there would be no danger even so if our bodies really became useless as a means of communication and we transferred totally to the learned verbal symbols of speech. We give up screams, crying, grunts, and other nonverbal sounds except at times of great emotional stress. We continue, however, to express our feelings in our bodies, largely because this is outside of our awareness. As Dr. Plant has said,

> Verbal modes of expression lend themselves to the intellectual processes whereas what one calls the psychomotor tensions are the modes of emotional expression.

At the end of a day when we have had to spend a number of hours in intense thinking, we are aware of pain and tension in the back of our necks. Again, on a day when the children in the family or the schoolroom have been more than usually demanding, noisy or quarrelsome, we will probably feel physical weariness throughout our whole body and be vaguely aware of tension in the muscles of our face. We may even be aware of a tick at the side of our eyes or a tightening of our jaw. Will we also be aware of the many expressions of frustration, anger and defeat that we have been revealing in myriads of ways and more and more clearly as the day progressed, no matter what words we may have been using? Similarly, in moments of excitement or happiness, we restrain ourselves from any physical expression of our feelings except with our most intimate friends or family. Yet, according to John Martin,

> Nature has so constituted us that movement is the medium in which we live our lives.

As I have worked in the field of dance as a means of direct communication through the past several years with a growing alertness to the expression of emotion in body action, I have been amazed at the disparity between words and action in the majority of people. We have centred so completely on verbal symbols that the communication in action passes unnoticed by the majority of people. At times I become fascinated hearing and watching two dissimilar conversations occurring simultaneously among people living and functioning in the normal world. Among mental patients there is apt to be less disparity.

Fortunately, in this restricted culture of ours, there is a medium of expression for us to use which is built out of our natural need to communicate with body action. In the dance, freedom of action is demanded and is socially acceptable. Many other aspects of dancing are very important and are more frequently discussed, however. Dancing is valuable as a group activity, as a tool for poise in social situations, a means of developing body co-ordination, posture, and above all as fun. Dance is sometimes called the matrix of the arts and can be very useful in aiding a child to develop an appreciation of music as well as an awareness of music forms and dynamics, or a sense of line and form in drawing and modelling. It is possible to encompass the arts and show the usefulness of dance as adjunctive to each.

These attributes are often stressed in a discussion of dance with a too frequent neglect of the role which is of major importance to the child. Education is basically for the devlopment of a body of intellectual knowledge from which to reach out in specific areas in proportion to an individual's curiosity and comprehension, as well as the learned skills related to this body of knowledge. It is unfortunate that as a person develops in the use of verbal symbols and the academic learning acquired through their use that his ability to express emotion is often conversely repressed to the vanishing point. This is doubly unfortunate when it is unnecessary.

In many cultures throughout the world, dancing is still a part of the cultural pattern of the community. When this is true you will also see strong physical action being used to accompany the words which are being spoken. Facial expression, arms, hands, the whole body come strongly into play so that the total person is involved in what is going on. Much of the insecurity that is felt in our culture might be alleviated if we gave more free expression to our feelings and accompanied our words with appropriate expression in our bodies.

Children have a limited vocabulary at best for many years. They are still to a large extent dependent on their natural modes of expression. It is during this period of transition that they are forced to restrain their natural impulse to use action rather than words. Dance, then, can be a useful tool to avoid the feeling of isolation that is so prevalent among the majority of people. If, as the young woman at the hospital stated, we could start dancing at three or four—or rather continue to dance after three or four until we are too old to move perhaps we would not find it so difficult to let others know what we feel when we are with them. We would know where to find them.

One of the assets of the person who is mentally ill, or the child who is disturbed is that he is able to express his feelings in movement and action. This is often frightening to others, not because this is basically wrong, but because of the strange code of almost immobile social behavior. It is really good to be able to know immediately what a person is feeling as well as what he is thinking. Then one has a feeling of meeting and knowing the total person.

Expression of feeling in body action, whether in natural ways or in dance action does not lead to unrestrained, chaotic action, nor does it lead to uncontrolled "acting out". Quite the contrary is true. One needs only to participate in a dance session with a group of emotionally upset people to know that this is the case. It is after a dance session at the hospital, not before, that one is aware of relaxation, use of verbal speech in a free way, and a warmth of companionship among the participants. This is true not because they are patients, but because they are people.

Because dance is not a spontaneous part of the community life, it should be a part of the cultural training of all children, so that they may retain a sense of a total person participating with others. Dance is not an extra frippery. It is rather a real essential to the educational and cultural growth of the child.

Some Observations on the Psychodrama Sessions at Chestnut Lodge

Reprinted courtesy of Chestnut Lodge from *Eighth Annual Chestnut Lodge Symposium.* Rockville, Maryland, November 9, 1962. Pp. 19-31.

with JUDITH R. BUNNEY

A free form of psychodrama was started at Chestnut Lodge a number of years ago. It was felt that this form of group action could be used within the particular setting of the Lodge and not be out of place. At first it was called spontaneous drama to distinguish it from other forms of psychodrama, including the techniques of Dr. Moreno. However, after a very short time, people in general were calling these sessions psychodrama. We shrugged and stopped using the term "spontaneous drama".

At first, it was the intention of the Lodge to include in the group only staff and personnel for a better understanding of the interaction between members of the staff and between patients and staff. At that time, the members of the group assumed the roles of patients when scenes involved patients.

This form of structuring of the sessions was continued for about two years. At the request of a group of patients, it was decided to try a pilot project on Hilltop II which would include in the group both patients and personnel.

At the time that the Center was opened, the decision was made to include any Lodge patient who wished to attend the sessions.

However, the general structure of these sessions, as well as the goals, has remained the same throughout the several phases. It has always been the intention of the leader to create an environment in which free discussions of interaction between people on a realistic level can develop. Through the lack of pressure from the leader the members of the group seem able to become involved with one another in a supportive way. Often antagonisms between individuals develop, but even then they seem to feel sufficiently secure to continue communication.

This is vastly different from the structure used by the majority of psychodramatists. An essential part of their techniques is a very positive control. Players who are called auxilliary egos retain a given attitude and keep the scene within an established and often a pre-established structure.

Auxilliary egos or supportive players aid in the development of scenes here, but they are not pre-established. A patient who has presented a problem will suggest the people whom he feels can give him support, or some of the group will ask to enact the scene when they emphathize with the problem as it was presented.

Too often the frustration of the so-called "star", with established auxilliary egos, will lead him to speak at greater length than he originally intended. In the free-form style, scenes can cut or be augmented as the group wishes. The scene can also be cut at the discretion of the leader.

In spite of the fact that scenes are structured around specific problems of functioning in relationships on a day-to-day basis, the discussion centers around emotions involved in these relationships which are frightening to the members of the group.

Quite logically, among the subjects which create the greatest excitement, involvement, and tension are the emotions surrounding or resulting from aggressiveness, violence or fear and the danger of the inability to control them. Actually, it seems that no subject is considered that does not have fear as a large component of the feeling tone.

Through the free but broadly controlled structure of the sessions the patients are able to come forth with their own specific needs and frustrations rather than those suggested by the leader. They often speak of situations where they have felt a lack and a need. A great bitterness seems to accompany many of their statements of the deprivation of things which they feel within themselves. Nevertheless, no conclusion is reached in the psychodrama session.

Reports have been made of more than 90 psychodrama sessions over a period of more than two years. In reviewing these reports it has been interesting to note that there is a consistent repetition of certain feelings expressed by the group, regardless of the change of membership. The most recurrent problem dealt with at psychodrama is the complex of anger, hostility, violence and control, which was the focus at 13 sessions. We were surprised to learn that the next most frequent topic was warmth, love and marriage and lack of possibility of experiencing these. Hopelessness and worthlessness were discussed very often and then, in order of frequency, came sex, and loneliness. Other themes that came up repeatedly were isolation, authority, rejection, leaving Chestnut Lodge, which included fear of facing the world, and the question of the purpose of psychodrama. These subjects take different paths according to the way they are presented, and the group that is present.

Again, in reviewing the reports of the sessions, an interesting pattern emerges. Prior to scenes where the group is concerned with intense and frightening emotions, tension seems to be building. During this period they can talk only of superficial things: money, big business or anything far removed from human feelings. Suddenly someone will speak of a personal problem.

At one session, when the group centered on the expression of feelings of anger, together with the fear and guilt aroused by this, one of the group members suddenly addressed me "You people can express anger about a specific thing and then turn it off. We are afraid of doing that for fear our whole fountain of hostility will burst forth and everything will be destroyed".

Following sessions involved with expressions of intense feeling, the topics are neutral ones with little excitement. Escorting and privileges are sometimes discussed, together with patients' feelings about these. Not surprisingly, these feelings are stated in a very mild fashion. Reflections of ward meetings, functioning as an outpatient, hospital policy or other non-threatening subjects that are under general discussion throughout the Lodge may also be brought to the sessions at this time.

The goals of psychodrama sessions are twofold. One is to enable a group of patients to share their feelings with one another. In this way, they can often feel less of their usual isolation. The second goal is for the group to try to see more clearly what they are really saying in presenting a problem. Consequently, there must be no demand, or seduction to speak of more completely than a person wishes at a given moment. By permitting the group to be supportive to the person speaking, rather than having the leader stimulate the discussion too far in one direction, people can come forth with very real feelings which may open the door to further discussion but not resolve a given problem. The patient group seems to be clear about these goals; even though discussion of them is presented at intervals.

In one session they clearly stated that the purpose of the sessions is to view problems from different angles, rather than to work through the problems. Occasionally, however, patients will be very frustrated about psychodrama and will say many negative things about it. Yet, when they have some need of the kind to be enacted or shared in discussion with the group, they will return and either be supportive to somebody else or bring a problem of their own into the session.

Although psychodrama sessions are not directed in an authoritarian way, there seems to be no confusion in the various participant roles. Miss Chace is accepted as the leader when she is present, and the group accepts Mrs. Bunney in this role at the occasional sessions when Miss Chace is absent. Although remaining in a neutral, non-directive role, an occasional work, recognition of a given patient, or the structuring of a scene when the discussion indicates a readiness for this. Only through confidence that the leader has control of the situation can the group be creative and express feelings freely. Consequently, the group calls on her only occasionally to assume the role of authority.

Mrs. Bunney, as a staff member consistently supportive to the group and to the leader, sometimes speaks for the group, sometimes structures a scene and sometimes enters the discussion. Occasionally she is chosen by a patient to participate in a scene. This usually happens when the role called for is one of authority.

The roles which the patients assume differ at different times, both in relative positions of authority and in person involvement. The patient leader, who may remain a leader for several sessions is someone who presents a problem that stimulates the interest of the group.

Although the problem presented may seem to be a personal one, it is actually one with which the members of the group can empathize. However, the group will not tolerate a problem presented on a superficial level. They have several ways of handling this irritation. Non-participation in the discussion or leaving the group, as they are always free to do, are the two most effective ways. Each patient leader seems to have his group of patient participants. They are interested and supportive in the discussions, and usually become involved in the scenes. Some of these patients are very obvious and verbal in their involvement while others choose to be supportive by implication, or by an occasional verbal comment.

Discussions are not always viewed from equally honest viewponts. Sometimes they will be presented with a great deal of superficiality, sometimes with a great deal of defensiveness, but sometimes with an amazing amount of honesty. However, it is usual for one of the patients who speaks in symbolic terms to cut through conversation that is too superficial with a very direct comment. Frequently, this will stop useless discussion and cause the group to speak more directly. The meaning is usually quite clear, although the terms in which the person speaks are obscure.

While psychodrama is essentially a verbal transaction, many nonverbal patients or patients who are unable to express themselves clearly attend, and are an integral part of the sessions. In reviewing the sessions, it is clear how interested the verbal patients are in these non-verbal patients, wanting them to express an opinion, asking them for a statement or being alert to their non-verbal communications. Much attention and tolerance is given to them when they do make an attempt to participate with a sudden sound or movement. The evening that one of them spoke to us of her reasons for her manner of functioning, was a startling example. People responded and included her in the group. Since then she has acted out by walking through the scenes and doing other things that the group ordinarily would not tolerate. Somehow they allow her this privilege without interfering with her behavior.

The group has less tolerance for the overly verbal patient who talks too much about purely personal affairs and consequently fails to involve the group. The group is also extremely impatient when someone is purposefully disrupting or avoids real feelings by holding forth on philosophical contemplation of emotion. On the contrary, they accept someone who has a pressing problem and takes over the group for an overlong period of time for the purpose of somehow organizing himself to the point of being able to express some of his feelings.

In general, the patients have carte blanche. They are allowed to set the scene, structure it, and choose the people with whom they wish to participate. If they are unable to do this, Miss Chace, as leader, offers suggestions. However, the direction the scene is to take is never dictated. People get involved in the scenes and, as one staff member has described it, what is said is intensely real; actual feelings come out, and there is nothing artificial to hide behind. Consequently, the scenes sometimes take surprising turns. At times Miss Chace uses the "alter ego" and at others the "role reversal" techniques when the scene is not able to move forward in the usual manner. The people are asked to switch roles, and to play the scene from the other side of the fence.

A typical evening of psychodrama starts with a circle of chairs being arranged by one of the patients or an aide in the Activities Center. People come in as people, not as patients or staff, and sit informally in the circle. Coffee is served, and a discussion usually begins naturally without much encouragement. The tone of these meetings varies greatly. Sometimes it is a silent group, sometimes the group immediately organizes itself for discussion; at other times there are small separate groups casually talking, or there are confusing elements when people try to cause interference.

Gradually the discussion focuses on one topic which perhaps will develop into a scene if there are enough people who empathize with the problem or the topic is suitable for action. It is always hoped that when the discussion formalizes a scene or scenes will develop so that the feeling expressed in the discussion can be viewed and clarified on an action level.

Starting from some simple question, the actual subject emerges as a phase of an intense, frustrating emotion, which is related in the scene to some incident in which a specific patient is involved.

One of the group will say, "How do you handle feelings of anger expressed to you?" or, "How do you apply for a job?" or, "How do you feel at home in a social situation?" Such discussions usually involve the majority of people present.

Scenes take place in the center of the circle of patients without the benefit of lighting effects or staging. Chairs serve as all manner of props, from cars to beds. The scene usually develops in such a way that the essential aspects of the problem can be viewed. The group can then discuss what went on with a chance for both the patient leader and the others to feel an emotional response. They also comment on whether or not the scene was real. The role players also are able to say how they felt in the scene. Often this discussion period takes much longer than the actual scene itself, as they look at what was actually going on between people, not only in the action but within the group as a whole.

There are times when a patient first presents a problem for discussion at one session, then moves on to participate in scenes with action at another session and finally progresses to group activity outside of psychodrama.

On a very cold night in February, a patient, Mr. R., came to the psychodrama session, arriving as it was in progress. He is described in the report as being very tight-lipped and having great difficulty in speaking. He stated that his feelings made him wish to kill people involved with him. He also stated that he felt hopeless and that he was incurable. Five different people entered into this discussion with him, and one said: "Why do you have to feel this way? It bothers me very much when you say that."

Since the group was interested and attentive, Mr. R. developed his feelings. He revealed more and more of his plan to injure another patient. He described in more detail his plan to hit this person with a steel chair, which would paralyze him. "There's no turning back, really! I know this must be done". Miss Chace said, "Perhaps you are asking for some help about this," and he replied, "The way you can help me is by handing me one of those steel chairs". The discussion ended with more of Mr. R's hopeless feelings.

He did not carry out his aggressive plan, and returned to the group the following week. He was welcomed, and he stated that he wondered if we had been talking about him. Miss Chace responded that we had not been doing so and that our topic had been the difficulty involved in the giving and receiving of compliments. He began to tell us how he had been down at the pond and had been feeling extremely lonely. He stated that he had been smoking a great many cigarettes, began feeling confused as he walked back and thought he would stop psychodrama session. He felt that he was going "out of contact," and that a person should seek the company of people who could recognize him as an individual when this happens. Then, possibly, he would not have the need to go off into the "wild blue yonder." He had come to psychodrama because, previously, he had been able to speak to the group. Another quite disturbed patient entered into the discussion telling of her own experiences of becoming withdrawn. Other patients questioned them both, and the report states, "Everyone seemed extremely involved and very interested, not curious, but really interested in the experience and feelings of the people talking."

On the following week, Mr. R. came to the session again, and was able to contribute to the general subject, competition, which was brought up by another patient. A scene was structured in which he was able to paticipate in a supporting role. However, he commented that the role he was playing was not his usual manner of behaving.

Outside of the session, he mentioned how appreciative he was of the interest and support he had received at psychodrama the week before. The next week it was reported that Mr. R. wanted very much to come to psychodrama. However, he did not join the group as he was chairman of decoraticns for the Mardi Gras party, and was in the midst of the group which was working on this!

There are times when his usual way of functioning blocks a patient even when he wishes to present a problem at psychodrama. If it is sufficiently pressing, however, he will continue to bring his problem to the sessions until he is able to speak to the group.

On the first presentation Mr. P. tried to discuss his feelings of responsibility for things that had happened to a great many people. A scene was structured for him to talk to a friend on a long distance call. However, he was unable to respond with warmth or interest to the patient playing his friend. The group felt that he was unable to hear them as they talked to him about this and the scene was closed.

Six weeks later, Mr. P. was able to bring his problem to the session again. He jumped on a table wildly waving his arms to gain attention and spoke in a loud voice about his feelings of inadequacy and inferiority. He demanded that he be declared unworthy and therefore a person to be killed. The group felt that he wanted them to enact a trial scene. This was structured with the group acting as a jury.

During the trial Mr. P spoke to the ghost of his father. Although the father is living, the group accepted Mr. P's feeling about him. The father assured Mr. P. that he felt as a father toward him and was proud of many of his achievements. The jury dismissed the charges, stating that it was Mr. P's own feelings about himself that made him feel an inferior person and that perhaps he could do something to bring about a change. They stated that other people did not consider him worthy of being killed. Mr. P seemed relaxed, but most interesting was the solid group integration and support of him.

There are some patients who are very regular in their attendance at the psychodrama sessions. This roles vary from merely entering into the discussion periods to presenting a problem and becoming the patient leader. Mrs. C. is one of these members of the group.

On one particular evening she seemed very distressed and stated that she was too restless to stay for more than a few minutes. Her manner encouraged the members of the group to speak and someone commented "It sounds as though you have been very low", she responded, "Low isn't even the word". She then began to speak of her feelings of worthlessness and hostility towards others. Mrs. C. had great difficulty in expressing her feelings of guilt because of her inability to rid the world of herself, wringing her hands, lowering her head and crying. She expresed the feeling that she was in the way of everyone. She was asked how people could help her to feel their warmth toward her. A scene was structured where she was to try to reach another patient in the role of a person feeling depressed and alone. She was unable to reach out and a new scene was structured where Mrs. C. played herself. She was able to permit the supportive player to reach her side, but could not tolerate her remaining. Mrs. C. spoke angrily, saying "Just get out of my room and leave me alone." The supportive player felt that she had functioned on a feeling rather than a word level as she approached Mrs. C.

Mrs. C. was visibly relaxed after the scene and was able to enter the discussion, acknowledging that she felt such hostility towards others that she had difficulty in acknowledging friendship or warmth expressed to her. The group continued to discuss anger, hostility and hopelessness for the remainder of the session and lingered after the usual time for ending the session.

As the previous scenes indicate, the major purpose of the psychodrama sessions seems to be that of creating a climate in which patients can express intense emotions of even the most negative kind and yet experience a feeling of sharing with others. Even though the focus of the evening is on a feeling that frequently causes isolation from others, the interaction between members of the group is usually a warm and positive one. Scenes and discussions were chosen which could show this aspect of the sessions.

However, as previously stated, there are an equal number of sessions which deal with the desires of the people involved for love, marriage and friendship. Even here, however, a great deal of support comes from the group and is essential, as the problem is always that of the fear of a close relationship or fear of the inability to experience emotions with others because of a feeling of unworthiness.

It has been impossible in this paper to give in detail the group discussions which enable the patient to see his problems from other points of view. Again let me stress that these discussions are left open ended, thus leaving the patient with an open door for discussion where the problem can be resolved with the therapist.

The Structuring of Dance Session for Varying Needs of Patients

Reprinted courtesy of the National Association for Music Therapy, Inc., from *Music Therapy*, 12 (1962), pp. 63-68.

From past experience in speaking to music therapists about dance in institutions, I have become aware that people are often under the impression that I always conduct sessions in the manner in which I lead them with the very withdrawn and regressed groups. I feel that this is natural, as these are the groups about which I speak most frequently. They are composed of people who are the most difficult to reach in any way, or with whom one rarely can form even a tenuous relationship. However, there are many other people in the hospital who can gain great satisfaction through working in groups or individually in dance or body action for communication and emotional release. While the same principles hold true, the actual structure of the specific sessions is very different in various areas of the hospital.

Today, the problem is not only one of assisting with patients who will stay in the hospital indefinitely, but in structuring dance sessons to give support to the people who are making an all-out drive to leave, or to keep from having to seek the care within it. When I speak of indefinite periods of time for staying in the therapeutic community, I am referring to those who come because of an acute break, whose stay may be a very short one, from a matter of a few weeks' time to six months or a year, as well as to those whose stay may be a matter of years or even a lifetime. These patients will be part of the hospital community for some time to come, and, consequently, they take a great deal of the time of the hospital staff.

Today, with the new attitudes and new help from many directions, the interchange between the hospital and the community, new drugs for assisting patients in functioning, and the need to reduce the population of the ever-growing large hospitals, changes in approach must be sought by all members of the staff. This means changes in the structuring of dance sessions as well as nursing care and the other ancillary services.

Day-care clinics are a usual part of large hospitals today. The people who remain at home, but who are having difficulty surviving the pressures of daily living, are the citizens of these clinics. It would be pointless to have the care of these patients or his return home would be on the basis of having permanent care by the family. Fortunate, in the midst of his misfortune, was the child whose family could afford to send him to a special school where his needs in growth were cared for as well as those caused by his illness. Within the past ten years the attempt has been made, often inadequately, to change this gloomy outlook for the child who becomes ill. Today, child centers within the hospital setting are being established. These range from areas where the child lives on a 24-hour basis to day treatment centers which provide school programs, therapy, and other activities geared to his needs while he continues to live in a ward with adult patients. I am not speaking here of the many different clinics, special schools, and remedial education centers, but only of the large adult hospital which accepts the child for treatment.

Dance sessions in many or all of these settings, whether the large hospital or the small clinic, should contain the same elements. These are not too different in overall structure from creative dance sessions in any community. Opportunity should be given to the child to have subjective expression, learning about his own body in its motor functioning, new coordinating skills, growth in poise and self-control, and awareness of music in its rhythm and tonal sound.

The difference between the classes in the community and in the clinic or hospital setting lies in the goals of the leader and his awareness of the great variety of special needs on an emotional and functioning level of the different children. These needs will have little compatibility with the child's chronological age. The leader must be aware especially or the emotional age level at which the child is functioning. Then, and only then, can he supply the structure in body action into which the child can fit and from which he can gain some benefit. It is possible to furnish the child a group experience with his peers in spite of the many individual differences in ability and levels of functioning.

However, I am at a loss, personally, if I try to work with a group of children some of whom are emotionally disturbed and some of whom are brain damaged. One group needs rapidity of shift, as they are essentially over quick, and the other needs a slowness of approach and infinite patience in repetition of the action. It is my personal opinion that it is harmful to each group for them to be combined in joint sessions.

One important aspect of dance therapy is the conducting of sessions with individuals. The majority of sessions which I lead involve several patients, but there are a number of sessions each week with individual patients. These vary greatly in approach and method of leadership.

One interesting series of such sessions was with a schizophrenic boy of about fifteen years of age. He was a ward problem because he was very restless and overactive in spite of being essentially withdrawn from others. He was involved in considerable acting out, and in the course of this was often assaultive. Unfortunately, he would choose as his target student nurses and the nurse in charge of the ward.

I was asked by the clinical staff to attempt to make a contact with him in dance, and thus to enable him to express some of his anger through body action which might be useful to him. During the session he was permitted to choose his own music, and at first he was fascinated by pantomiming swordplay with me to a *paso doble* record. For weeks on a once-a-week basis he would ask for this music and repeat much that he had done in the previous session. However, after having danced the swordplay, which had obvious symbolic meaning to him, he would want soft music and, quite logically (from his point of view), he would want to be held like a baby and rocked. This I would not do, stating that he was not a baby and was quite capable of his own independent action. However, I would then do swinging and rocking movements with him while we were standing together.

Occasionally, he would accept joint endeavor in walking, running, or jumping. After expressing different basic emotions from the symbolic aggressiveness of the swordplay to rocking and then to more outgoing movement, he suddenly said one day: "It is good to express your feelings, but what do you say when people never say anything warm?" This was a realistic question, as his parents were both very rigid and anxious people who rarely expressed anything verbally, other than irritation with him for being ill or worry about his ever getting well. His mother substituted bringing him food for any expression of warmth of feeling, even though she often held him in her lap.

At one point not long after we had started working and after a forced absence on my part for two or three weeks, he became more withdrawn and mute on the ward. The staff was concerned about the necessity for tube-feeding him, as he was refusing to eat. He had expressed the fear that his food was poisoned. The staff felt that since I worked in the area of body action, it might be acceptable for me to try to eat with him. Lunches for both of us were served on the same plate and he accepted from me the food which I was eating. I did not spoon-feed him but would hand the food to him. He resumed eating in the dining room at the next meal.

Soon after this, he was assigned to a therapist from the psychology department. We agreed between us and with the ward psychiatrist to make the dance sessions a three-way session, to prevent rivalry, so that he could see that it was possible to relate to more than one person at a time. These sessions seemed to go well, and he used the dance to test one and then the other alternately. Occasionally, the three of us would have lunch together, and he would ask that we exchange food again—with obvious implications.

Through many ups and downs, he has gradually lessened his retreating from others. At one point he asked to do things with other boys in the way that they do things. His doctor felt that he was not yet ready for this, and consequently this new phase of activity was delayed temporarily. However, he is now working with a group of other boys; while his acceptance of them is still tentative, he seems to be able to join in their activity with a gradual lessening of anxiety.

The majority of individual sessions are on an entirely different level, however. These hours often are scheduled to enable one patient who finds it difficult to express emotion to use free and spontaneous dance action to say nonverbally those things he is unable to say when he is with others. Miss D., who is usually very constricted in her relationships with others and equally stereotyped in speech, was dancing recently with warmth and expansiveness. Another person, who was watching her, suddenly spoke. "Why, Miss D., you are a dancer. I don't think I have ever known who you really were before." This was an exciting moment for the person watching the dance which had such an impact on her, as she has spoken very rarely in the last two years.

Sometimes individual sessions are held for the purpose of developing body control with people who can tolerate a group only with extreme anxiety. In these instances, an attempt continually is being made to help the patient to accept others in functioning with her.

The final type of session which I am presenting will be with a group of people who are psychotic but who can communicate verbally, although with difficulty. Often they can talk about feelings and ideas while they are moving together. Their conversation will travel from talk of home, their feelings of neglect, frustration, and fear of inadequacy, to delusions of themselves in positions of importance or even religious identification. In presenting this kind of session I have attempted to structure it as a scene, since one of the difficulties of the person functioning in the world is a lack of spontaneity in response to stimuli which call for unstudied speech as well as unstudied movement. One of our assets is self-control, which keeps us in the thinking area with other people who are essentially strangers to us. Our failure is fear of nonconformity. One asset of the mentally ill patient is the ability to respond emotionally regardless of the situation. One of his failures is his fear of lack of ability to conform or control his emotions.

Therefore, the session will need to be structured and enacted. The two groups of people functon in different ways. In relating across the chasm in this area, one can only attempt to understand and empathize.

The Power of Movement with Others

Reprinted courtesy of *Dance Magazine*, 38 (June, 1964), pp. 42-45, 68

The leader in the field of Dance Therapy explains her m
with hospitalized mental patients

From man's earliest days on this earth down through the ages, dance has served as a means of communication with those suffering physical and mental disorders. The fact that even in the not-so-far past magical spirits were often deemed to be the culprits for illness, makes all the more logical the thought that the magic of dance was considered a potent healer.

Today, however, dance is being used more knowledgeably, in more structured ways, with recognition that properly used, it serves as handmaiden and colleague to medical specialists. In the area of mental and emotional illness there is no one who has brought more advancement to the field than the author of this article. At one time a member of the Denishawn Company, she has in recent years been Music and Dance Leader at Saint Elizabeths Hospital, Washington, D.C. and at Chestnut Lodge Sanitarium, Rockville, Maryland.

The article on these pages was prepared by Miss Chace, approved and presented to the members of the American Psychiatric Association at a meeting in Los Angeles a decade ago. It was not published by us at that time only because it was considered "specialists' " material and therefore not suitable for a dance publication. But the climate has changed considerably in recent years and Miss Chace agrees with us that there is a growing awareness and an intense interest in this phase of dance. She has therefore given us the privilege of printing, for the first time, this informed and fascinating report.

This article will be followed by another by Miss Chace, written especially for our readers. It will consider the requirements of personality and in training which today's therapist are required to have.

Lydia Joel

Introduction

Relation of dance movement to common modes of nonverbal communication.

Dance has been used by man since the beginning of civilization as a satisfactory means of communicating his feelings.

It is closely allied to the nonverbal forms of communication which everyone unconsciously uses together with the verbal, but on which the acutely ill mental patient who is inarticulate is almost totally dependent.

Our word-centered culture causes us to repress these more archaic ms of communication to the point where, as adults, we rarely are aware of our need to feel empathy through body movement and body contact. Dance, then, in this culture is especially important as supplying an acceptable means of meeting this basic need. This medium of communication is often used by people in the contemporary restricting environment as a means of relating to others and so preventing a feeling of isolation. There are case histories of people who remained out of hospitals until this means of expression was cut off from them. One of the contributing factors in the illness of Nijinsky was his deprivation in the dance.

Basic dance, then, either in group or as an individual expression, is especially well adapted for use as an adjunctive therapy of acutely ill psychotic patients, where communication is more restricted than among people in general.

Similarity of the bizarre and autistic posturings of the disturbed psychotic patients to accepted forms of dance in the contemporary concert dance.

The contemporary dance has consciously concerned itself with an attempt to understand the response of the body to inner emotions. It has also developed varying techniques to channel these movements into direct expression. The term "basic dance" has been coined to differentiate it from the artificial and elaborate forms of dance which depend upon physical "tours de force" as a means of entertainment, rather than communication.

The acutely ill, regressed schizophrenic patient, is largely cut off from the means of communication which are open to others in his environment. He makes use of body action to convey his emotions. Stripped of the usual repressions of our word-centered culture, he is able to use his body with extraordinary directness and clarity in dance forms which are often closely parallel to those of the modern dancer. Both groups make use of symbolization in body action. While the modern dancer uses them for communicating an idea to a participating audience, and the schizophrenic patient uses them for giving expression to autistic emotion, they both arrive at remarkably similar forms.

One young man used the entire floor space available to him in his day room to dance a formal processional. His body control was superb and there was no superfluous movement. His entire body was involved in stylized motions expressive of grandiose power. He alternated this with the most abject grief as he sank to the floor as if he wanted to bury himself in it. As he had not used verbal communication for many weeks, I was asked to dance with him, to form a relationship, if possible. At the time of our first meeting, I was convinced that he must have been a pupil of Harald Kreutzberg. Many of the gestures he used were identical with those of the German dancer. He accepted my dancing with him and after six or seven sessions, he spoke to me. He was able to tell me that he had never studied dancing in any form. At this time he spoke mostly of the delusion that he was God, which he alternated with expressions of deep hopelessness, as he had in his dance.

Similarly, Martha Graham, in her dance, *Lamentation*, might be any one of many patients wrapped in their blankets, absorbed in their deep withdrawal, who use movements almost identical with hers, to express their smothering guilt.

One characteristic of modern dance is its concern with the dancer in space. The schizophrenic patient by his very self-containment makes one aware of the space that he is not occupying. The manic-depressive patient makes extraordinary use of the space in which he moves. He withdraws from the environment or moves out into it with an acute awareness that seems to concern itself with space above and below his, as well as the plane on which he is moving. Any concert dancer might well envy him his mastery of this element in action. He seems aware of no limitation as he dances. He expresses his rapidly changing emotions with directness and clarity and in understandable terms.

Action Patterns:

The manic

As stated in the previous section, the person who is experiencing a manic phase of the manic-depressive psychosis uses body action effectively and directly either to augment his verbal communication or to reveal his underlying emotional response of the moment. This emotion often appears as one of hostility, which seems to be caused by his inability to achieve an answer to his needs of the moment as quickly as he wishes, or by a feeling of restraint from authority figures or restrictions of his environment. The quick, impatient movements, similar though exaggerated, to those anyone might use, and the need to move into space, even though someone or something is in the way, often causes needless retaliation. It has been my experience that patients use this aggressive behavior pattern as an expression of their feeling of the moment rather than toward an individual.

The ability to use movement as an expression of emotion in a direct way, together with his command of space about him, makes the manic patient an exciting and stimulating dancer. His movements are exaggerated, strong, beautifully coordinated dance motions, but they always appear like expressions of anger, destruction, and despair. He seems to have no mental image of himself as successful, but only as reaching, attacking, and then despairing, a result of his childhood history. When the dancer is left alone to complete his improvisation, he inevitably finishes it on the floor in a posture of self-degradation. Even though he physically tires himself, and in spite of the discharge of a great deal of emotional and physical energy, he seems to feel no relaxation. He continues to shout and is restless, with no lessening of difficulties with people in his environment.

During the process of re-socialization, this means of communication is gradually repressed until the patient moves with rigidity and overrestraint as he leaves the hospital. Miss H expressed this feeling by saying, "I have learned to suppress my real emotion, but in doing so, I have reinforced my basic guilt feelings."

Depressed psychotic

The patient who is lethargic and depressed is equally able to express his feelings through his movements and tone of voice. These actions are less exciting and stimulating than those of the opposite extreme, but are no less true in their expression. The posture, aloneness of response, apparent indifference to the environment, and refusal to participate in usual activities are all ways of expressing emotion which are far more direct than any words could convey.

Patients who are experiencing the slowed up state accompanying an emotional depression seem to be more aware of their body responses than the majority of mental patients. They seem to feel an added anxiety, caused by their inability to function in an accustomed way. They will frequently seek dance activity as a constructive means of alleviating their fright and bewilderment. The temporary relief afforded in feeling their bodies relaxed and stimulated seems to be important to them. Miss H was very aware of these feelings of lack of coordination, lethargy, and inability to concentrate when she was feeling upset emotionally. She would approach me directly, saying, "I can't make my body work. Please help me." At the end of a session of exercises for relaxation and coordination, she would say, "Thanks, now I can manage." She alternated between having lessons by herself and participating in group sessions when she was able to be with other people without a sense of inadequacy.

The patient who is expressing depression in restless activity seems to feel no reduction of his anxiety in these repetitive actions. Someone may walk twenty-four hours a day, wring hands, or rock in a chain constantly, but his body tensions seem to be as intense at the end of this time as at the beginning, even though there can be no doubt about the feelings being acted out. The initial response from people in the environment is usually one of sympathy and a wish to alleviate the patient's anxiety. However, when little response from the patient is elicited in attempts to distract him, the attitude of the environment often changes to one of hostility and resentment, and as a result, the patient feels further rejection.

If left to himself, or met on a purely verbal level, the patient will continue in this type of movement pattern for long periods of time.

However, he is often very responsive to movement in rhythm. He can be stimulated to move with a complete change of movement pattern, with an apparent easing of tensions to the point where he can enter into conversation, laugh, and join in group activity, even though on a temporary basis.

Schizophrenic

Members of the personnel of any mental hospital, from the physician to the psychiatric aide, are aware of the posturings of the schizophrenic patient. These patterns of movement are considered meaningful to the patient. It is rarely successful, however, to watch these action patterns in an attempt to feel with the patient and then translate this feeling into words, which in turn are difficult for the patient to follow.

One characteristic of the movement of the schizophrenic patient makes it seem more bizarre to the onlooker than perhaps it actually is. He seems to use only his hands, feet, and head to express his feelings. This creates movements which seem distorted to those of us who use our whole body. His withdrawal from the space about him also seems unnatural to us. Once one has accepted these two characteristics of his movements, however, he no longer seems strange and non-understandable. As one moves with him in his fashion rather than one's own, it is startling to discover how very direct he is being and how little he is making any attempt to hide his fear, guilt or hostility. An added factor brought into the picture in moving with a patient who is absorbed in fantasy is the predominant one of isolation. To speak of the isolation of an acutely ill schizophrenic patient becomes almost a cliché, but feel with a patient this removal in space is no cliché. It makes understandable his lack of any overt attempt to relate to those about him. He is unable to communicate his feelings in intelligible verbal terms and those about him are often either too repelled or made anxious by his direct communication in movement to attempt to understand.

He is also revealing through his movement his feelings of helplessness and dependence. It is not strange, then, that he seems to get no relief from anxiety through his posturings when he recieves no satisfactory answer from those about him, on a level which he can accept. He seems to be lost in a four-way dearth of communication. The patient is expressing himself verbally in ways which do not communicate for the most part, but saying things directly in ways which are ignored, while those about him are speaking verbally in ways which do not reach him and expressing feelings nonverbally of which they are unaware. Some of the bewilderment concerning people who are very sick must come from these four-way means of communication which never meet.

I think it is through the attempt to move with patients in forms similar to theirs that has caused many of them to say "You have known me from the beginning," and others to state "Nobody wants to be alone." These remarks say clearly "You answered me in movement when that was my speech."

Although the bizarre actions of mental patients are well recognized as protective mechanisms, they seem frequently to be ignored as attempts to communicate.

I believe dancing in symbolic forms for the schizophrenic patient has an important aspect, when it is a shared experience. Since these feelings of guilt, overdependency and loneliness are too overwhelming to put into verbal terms, but can be directly expressed in movement, it follows logically, that they must be answered satisfactorily to the patient to prevent further withdrawal into isolation.

Description of dance therapy sessions

Dance sessions at Saint Elizabeths Hospital and at Chestnut Lodge Sanitarium are held in wards of the hospital as well as in a room designed for the sessions. These are always conducted with sufficient freedom to permit group action to develop, although the first part of the session is designed to encourage individual autistic and bizarre, though, to the patient, meaningful movement patterns.

Sessions with individual patients.

In certain instances dance sessions are held with or for individual patients who seem to feel too much anxiety when they are with a group, or who wish to use the dance for improvisations in releasing their emotions.

No attempt is ever made to structure a setting designed to bring into the patient's awareness his major problems, which remain the psychiatrist's province. However, the psychotic patient makes use of these sessions in ways that give evidence of the power of movement with others to break into his isolation and to help him feel able to communicate more satisfactorily for himself.

Mr. B was very excited, restless and rapidly changing in mood. He seemed to find difficulty in relating to people generally, on any satisfactory basis. At times when he was disturbed, he would frequently fight with men and be so sarcastic and threatening to women that they would avoid him whenever possible. At other times when he was able to function in a more acceptable way, on the surface, he would effectively keep people at a distance by a supercilious manner.

As I entered his ward for a dance session, he met me with his usual hostile manner, and in a truculent tone asked if I expected him to participate in some activity. I replied, "Not necessarily, but if you like, you might use some of your energy in exercise." In a baiting tone of voice, he replied, "Let's see what it is like."

We sat on the floor facing each other for a traditional modern dance leg and torso stretch. He used this exercise to pull me until it hurt, seeming to take delight in an attempt to rip me apart. When I admitted I had had enough, instead of stopping, he asked, "Who's next?" in a far less belligerent tone. He followed this with constructive body control exercise, seemingly to accept me without the need for his usual patterns. Saying he was tired, he then asked for some quiet music for a short period. As he sat quietly beside the phonograph, he wept. I sat on the floor beside his chair, moving only to change records. After a short while he noticeably relaxed. After about ten minutes of listening to the music, he asked for popular dance music to which we might dance together. He danced and chatted in an easy manner. Later in the day, he was able to participate with others on the tennis court and in other activities.

Several weeks later, he thanked me for my "help" (his word) which had enabled him to feel confident on a visit home. This help had been solely one of meeting him on a movement level as he shifted from overt hostility through dependence to the normal role of his own age and intellectual level. However, for him this session was significant, and although we conversed on only the most casual of subject matter, he was able to establish a relationship through the dance movement.

For some time prior to leaving the sanitarium, he acted as my assistant in some sessions, and found opportunities to "help" others in the group in an unobtrusive way. Meanwhile, his intensive psychotherapy is, of course, continuing. The dance session had been valuable in establishing empathy at a time when he felt isolated from others.

Many times, an individual dance session will rather dramatically emphasize the transition from relating to one person to group acceptance. Miss A was receiving insulin sub-shock treatment. As I entered the treatment room with the phonograph and records for the purpose of playing restful music during the rest period, Miss A was making threatening advances toward the nurses. The physician in charge, who was familiar with the dance sessions, suggested that I dance with her. Although the space available was limited to an aisle between the beds, we danced furiously together. In this instance, I met her hostile movements of attack with similar ones. The patient danced all manner of assaults on me, playing the role of a child in a tantrum, stamping her feet and pounding her fists in direct attack, seemingly bent on destroying her partner in the dance. I responded with answering movements of hostility. However, Miss A never actually touched me, and her actions were always in rhythm to the music being played, as she pantomimed the battle. Later, after she had expended much energy in this way, I sank to the floor in simulated defeat. Miss A quietly returned to her bed, where her treatment was immediately terminated. Although she remained in the room for another hour, she was quiet, and occasionally asked for specific records.

Later in the day, on going to her ward for dancing, I suggested to the nurse that she be allowed to remain on the porch where she would have a feeling of space without too close contact with the group and complete freedom to use the music in her own way. However, she came immediately to the door and asked to join the group, saying, "Now, I can dance with you instead of against you."

Although prior to this she had danced during her ward sessions it has always been alone or with me. Following this experience, however, she remained a part of the group in feeling, even though occasionally she might improvise her own dances for short times. She never later referred to this session, although she would often state that I knew and understood her.

In individual sessions a relationship is established with the dance therapist through her response in various ways to the patient's emotional expressions in movement. No demands are made to accept more orthodox dance patterns. Verbal conversation during the periods described is almost impossible. In each instance the patient gives outward expression to his conflicts and hostilities and through answering movement feels sufficient answer, understanding, and acceptance to alter his behavior patterns with the dance therapist. Some tensions augmented by association with others seem to be sufficiently modified so that he seeks wider companionship during this activity. As Miss H has verbally expressed this feeling, "When I am aware of myself, I can be with others."

Sessions with groups.

Patients participate in dance sessions throughout their stay in the hospital. However, the dancing seems to have special meaning to them while they are acutely ill. At a time when many outlets are cut off, they find themselves involved in an activity with other people in which their anxieties are reduced rather than augmented. Group feeling begins to develop at this time, even while the contact is almost totally on a movement level.

Here in the same room are perhaps twenty or thirty people. The session starts with multiple contacts on an individual basis. Miss H is dancing, absorbed in her fantasy. She is making use of the music without regard for its color, although she is following the rhythmic pattern. As she moves rapidly about the room, there is no feeling that she is aware of outward space. Her feet barely make contact with the floor; her hands may reach outward, but not into space. She may stretch upward in a grandiose gesture, but it seems strangely disembodied. This creates a feeling of loneliness and removal accompanying whatever other emotions of hate, fear, or need may be the specific theme of her dance.

It would be almost impossible to reach this patient with words. She is absorbed in her own world and she is unable to hear with comprehension. However, it is possible to approach her with a dance that is similar in pattern to her own. The patient will accept another dancer even though the feeling of her isolation remains for a time. The therapist remains with the patient for short periods of time, with a gradual lengthening of these periods. Eventually, the patient usually looks at the other dancer with recognition. Then a quick "hello" with an answering smile establishes the beginning of a relationship.

Simultaneously Miss D may be dancing with strong, active movements throughout the room. Her movements are aggressive and hostile. She may alternate between demands for phonograph records and dancing with leaps onto benches or dropping to the floor. She readily accepts a fellow dancer, provided the dancer moves according to her pattern.

As previously stated, if no one also joined Miss D in this dance, it would inevitably end in defeat. In entering this dance drama I have found that my role seems to be that of antagonist. I find that care is needed to underplay enough so that I am not the dominant figure, but the one on whom the assault is being made. Care must also be taken at this point that Miss D does not accept a role of dependency, following leadership in a "good child" manner, for if this occurs, she will not be able to accept the group, but will continue to dance her own emotions of hostile drive toward ultimate defeat.

When this action reaches a successful conclusion for the patient, and I have been the one defeated, Miss D will then dance with intense buoyancy and shortly thereafter will accept others to form a group.

After this contact the patient will frequently stay with the session, verbalizing about activities in the room, choosing records, and joining other dancers in unison movement.

The descriptions of these dancers are approximately those of the many dancers in the room. If a group is to be developed the dance leader must move rapidly from one to another until there is a gradual change from totally autistic movements to more orthodox dance action. As this change begins to take place, dancing with others will be in small groups of three or four, sometimes with the leader included and sometimes not. Finally a large circle will form. The dancing becomes more rhythmic, with stamping, hand clapping in unison, and more total body involvement, and verbal expression develops.

It is during the dancing in the circle that the withdrawn, usually motionless patient, is drawn into the activity and will even be able to join in the verbal conversation which develops at this time.

Miss C danced her own improvisations for several sessions before she was able to join the group. On the day she joined the group she said, "I have been saying one thing. Now I am ready to talk with others about many things."

Occasionally, withdrawn patients may use the rhythmic action of the circular dance group as support while they continue to dance by themselves. Mrs. R is withdrawn from the other patients on her ward for the greater part of the time. She remains curled up in a corner of the room absorbed in her own feelings. Occasionally she is obviously responding to hallucinations. She is unable to tolerate close contact with the members of a dance session as yet.

However, as the dance begins to absorb the majority of patients on her ward, and group patterns begin to develop, Mrs. R follows these rhythmic patterns with her eyes, her face becomes relaxed, and she responds with body movement to what is happening in the room rather than to her voices.

Suddenly, after a large circle has been formed, she begins a rhythmic stamping movement of her feet which carries her around the room just outside of the circle of other dancers. As she stamps, she moves her shoulders forward with alternate sharp jerks, reaching with her arms as she chants, in time to the music, about her loneliness and isolation from others.

Recently she suddenly demanded, "Play that again. It is from 1920 or so." Asked if she knew the music, she stated, "It belongs to the time of my beginning." The music was repeated and she continued to dance throughout the session with unusual intensity. At the close of the hour she relaxed heavily in her chair and in response to the remark said as a question, "You are tired?" She answered, "Yes, I have just lived twenty years, and now I am here." For the first time she moved close to the other patients and chatted and laughed with them as they returned to their wards.

The group dance sessions, even on the wards of acutely ill psychotic patients always progress from individual dancing in patterns expressive of emotional conflict to unison group movement accompanied by easy conversation and laughter. As previously stated, patients' own explanation of this phenomenon is that when they become aware of themselves they can then accept others.

Through group sessions in dance an individual is enabled to move from expressions of autistic emotional feelings, through the relating to others on a basic level compatible with her own, to acceptance of a group on a more adult level. Consequently, sessions in the dance are often the first steps toward participation in other forms of individual or group therapy.

Summary

Dance theapy, in making use of the basic form of communication, offers the individual a means of relating to the environment or to other people when he is cut off in the majority of areas of communication by the patterns of his illness. Contrariwise it offers an acceptable medium for a member of the personnel to discard the customary or verbal communication without embarrassment to himself or to the patient with the possibility of meeting on a level common to them both.

A patient's movements, meaningful to him, though bizarre, become understandable and acceptable to others as people relate to him by means of dance patterns. In proportion to the degree of acceptance from others that he feels, he seems able to accept himself with a concomitant reduction of his feeling of isolation and guilt. He can put aside temporarily, defense mechanisms to an increasing degree. This, in turn, seems to enable him to relate to a group and function within it in a manner that is satisfying both to the patient himself and to others. As the patient becomes more aware of himself as an entity functioning with other entities in comparative safety, verbal communication replaces the more basic ones and interest in his environment is widened. Fear of others is lessened and overdependence is reduced, so that he feels less need for protection and withdrawal from the environment.

Group interaction which begins to develop on a movement level in dance sessions has a definite continuing value as patients participate in other forms of individual or group therapy. In addition to its value as a means of initial contact through basic communication, it is valuable as a continuing group activity, toward which patients have an attitude that it is a home base where they can continue to release emotional energy.

Basic dance, either in group or as an individual expression, is especially well adapted for use as an adjunctive therapy on wards of acutely ill psychotic patients.

Dance Alone Is Not Enough . . .

Reprinted courtesy of *Dance Magazine*, 38 (July, 1964), pp. 46-47, 58.

Today's dance therapy demands special skills and training

Dance therapy is an exciting discipline that offers many satisfactions. Not the least of these is seeing eyes light up when a person who has shown little interest in what is going on suddenly becomes an interested person involved with others. It is the skill of the dance therapist, moving with intention, that has made this possible, that has stimulated this response.

Dance as such is used in many forms in clinics, special schools and institutions of all kinds for people with emotional difficulties. No recreation program is complete without parties centered around social dancing, square dancing and folk dancing. Classes in several forms of dance may be part of the program. Occupational therapists and physical therapists sometimes use dance with specific groups of patients for a particular purpose. Many music therapists use dance as a part of their music programs with groups or with individuals. But distinction must be made between the goals of these different uses of the dance and the training of the leaders. They need not to be the same. There is therapeutic dance, dance therapy or just dance, depending upon the needs of the participants, the particular setting, the goals of the leaders, and the leader's comprehension of *what* she is trying to accomplish, *how*, and *why*.

Everyone communicates on two levels, verbal interchange for thinking and nonverbal for relating with empathy and emotional expression. Dance as an aid for the release of emotions is as old as the establishment of communities of men. Tribal leaders used it in the rites of primitive society, and its use has continued, in one form or another, through the centuries.

Today, the teacher of dance in our lonely cities has more pupils who are seeking personal gratification than those with talent and ability who are working to develop into professional performers. People who seek dance and find healthy satisfaction in it are often those who find it difficult to relate to others on the usual levels. Expressing ideas and feeling in dance, and developing skill in dance action, gives them great personal satisfaction.

What is dance therapy?

In the usual dance class, the pupils are able to reach out to others in the class as much or as little as they wish, in a more or less adequate way, and still find what they seek. However, people who are so defeated in human relationships that they need professional help in a therapeutic setting require more support than they can find in a class where everyone makes use of the session for his own need and very possibly ignores others in the class.

Dance therapy is a specific use of rhythmic body action employed as a tool in the rehabilitation of patients in present-day institutions. While it makes use of those elements in dance which have caused it to be helpful at all times to all men, dance therapy is a purposeful and knowledgeable use of expressive action as a potent means of direct communication.

While both are working with rhythmic body action, the dance therapist is a group leader rather than a teacher. The dance therapist combines verbal and non-verbal communication to enable a patient to express feeling, to participate in human relationships, to increase prsonal self-esteem, to develop a more realistic concept of his body image, and through all of these to achieve some feeling of relaxation and enjoyment. Direct communication must happen continuously between the group and the leader. If this happens, a strong and useful relationship will develop between the leader and the patient; and from there between the patient and others in the group.

Demands on the therapist

The dance therapist is not teaching dance in order to develop performing artists, but is using her technical skills and her personal creativity and spontaneity to enable people to become more aware of themselves on a human, realistic level. In order for her to dare to work in terms of basic communication in body action, she must have resources sufficiently rich so that she can dare to free herself from specific technical forms.

The sessions must always be conducted in realistic and simple action. This requires a wide background in all dance forms, not only to understand what the patient is expressing in movement, but also to understand her own reactions and what she is expressing in answer to the patient. If she has an inadequate background in dance, or is bound by a specific technique, she will be unable to respond freely and spontaneously in a kind of direct communication far more rapid and volatile than the verbal level.

We are a word-centered culture, and we sometimes ignore the things we are saying directly with our body action. Patients are more aware of expressions of feeling from other people than many of us are. The leader must realize that there can be nothing artificial about her responses.

Few patients are skilled dance performers but many can express, through naturalistic movements, great intensity of feeling, using valid, though often unfamiliar, rhythmic patterns. The leader must be sufficiently free to accept these forms as creative expression and real communication on a human level. Therefore, it is important that she be aware of her own feeling in response to emotional expression from others. She cannot reject expressions of feeling because she is threatened by them. She must answer satisfactorily or the patient will be aware of her rejection, and she will augment the patient's isolation rather than reduce it. Many expressions of feeling which the leader will receive will be hostile, and she must be able to answer with her own movements so that it becomes a shared experience and thus modifies the emotion of the patient.

As a rule, dance therapy sessions are held in group. This means that numerous people are involved in a response to what is going on. No time can be spent in deciding what movements should be used to build the rhythmic action and interchange of the group. If the movements used are basically rhythmic and true in emotional expression, strong group But no amount of training will be of any use unless there is within the group. There will be people who are very withdrawn, others who are aggressive and hostile, and still others who are interested in being cooperative members of the group. The leader must relate to each of them in appropriate ways and help to make each of them able to function successfully.

Hostility must be released and accepted, fear of lonelines must be changed to a confidence in self and, ideally, the whole group works together with enjoyment while verbal conversation develops.

Qualities and training

Obviously, the dance therapist must have special training in order to make use of so vital and direct a means of relating. She must know what to do, and why, for people who have withdrawn from most human contacts. But no amount of trainig will be of any use unless there is within the person the sensitivity, creative spontaneity, and freedom of expression essential to the process of dance therapy.

It is impossible to be sure of what is going on in a session without learning to be aware of the meaning of communicative body action. The therapist must understand the basic difficulties of the patients and be able to empathize without identification. In other words, she must know what to do to relate to a patient's non-verbal expression in order to understand, but she must not become absorbed in it.

The training of the dance therapist must be as complete as it is for any of the other disciplines within a hospital, special school or clinic setting. She must be able to communicate with members of the other disciplines with mutual understanding. She must have her co-workers' confidence in her ability to function with patients in a useful and therapeutic way as part of the team and to use communication in body action in a knowledgeable way. Her role is as well defined as that of the nurse, the psychiatrist or a member of any of the other disciplines. When she understands her role, she can then be a part of the rehabilitation team.

Since dance therapy is a new profession, formalized standards have not yet been firmly established, but young people wishing to make a career of dance therapy must understand that it is a profession and as such requires as much training as other professions.

Academically, the dance therapist must have had courses in basic psychology, abnormal psychology, child development, group dynamics, group leadership, cultural anthropology, kinesiology and body mechanics. This should be in addition to continuing study within her specific field. She should have courses in choreography, music theory, art appreciation and dance, dance and more dance in many established forms. There is so much ground to cover that some people feel that the clinical training described below should be on the post-graduate level.

Unfortunately, although a growing interest is being shown in establishing degrees in dance therapy by several colleges and universities, I know of none which has yet done so. For the present, it is possible that programs leading to degrees in other forms of dance can be augmented.

Clinical background

And, in addition to such related academic training, there should a period of clinical training of not less than six months and preferably a year. Clinical training consists of participating in dance sessions with patients of varying degrees of illness under the close supervision of a professional dance therapist, attendance at clinical conferences with interns from other disciplines, and participation in other phases of training offered at a qualified training center. One extremely valuable training tool at St. Elizabeths Hospital is the participation of the dance therapist as a member of a group, along with other professional trainees under the leadership of a psychiatrist, in which each discovers a respective role and way of functioning in a group setting.

Yes, the trainee must not only become adept in using her own tool, but she must also develop in attitudes and modes of functioning in a way acceptable to the other disciplines. She must learn to understand the roles of the physician, the nurse, the psychologist and those who work in other therapies—and then her own role in relation to them. She will do well to absorb all of this within a year.

Summary

As a result of this initial training, successfully completed, the dancer will have developed 1) an understanding of the emotional functioning of mental patients; 2) an awareness of the meaning of communication in body action; and 3) a knowledge of where it is useful in the therapeutic setting as a part of the total treatment program.

Dancing for communication is also a very useful tool in the school or institution for the mentally or emotionally retarded child. Here the dance leader should have additional training in the knowledge of how such a child functions, what his assets and limitations are, as well as how his physical coordination relates to his mental abilities. Only with this knowledge can the dance therapist, working on a nonverbal level, be an aid to the other therapists and teachers in giving confidence and control to the child. When the leader has such training, dance can reach many children who find the use of words a difficult task, children who are frustrated in being understood, and who often lack emotional control.

Further specialized knowledge should also be acquired if the dancer wishes to do dance therapy with the physically handicapped, whether they are blind, deaf, hard of hearing or people afflicted with cerebral palsy or other related difficulties. Again, however, if you are speaking of dance therapy, you are speaking of the dance leader who is a professionally trained person who knows whether she is being helpful or not to the people with whom she is working and who can take guidance or supervision in a knowledgeable way from the medical or teaching staff. In other words, she has a framework from which to function that is compatible with the other disciplines.

There is a growing interest in research in the area of non-verbal communication. Again, there is need for training in the proper tools for research. The person must know what the methodology of research involves. It is possible to learn the needs of a person doing a research project and contribute those things which he needs. But, again, the dance therapist must have training in order to speak and function intelligently. *Dance alone is not enough in any phase of dance therapy.*

Given a more rounded background, what the dancer then does with her own medium is impossible to describe. With both formal education and specialized training as her framework, she can use her own sensitivity, creativity, and ability to communicate spontaneously through body action to add the dimension that must come from her and that is uniquely hers.

Many good and useful dance programs are today being conducted by volunteers and others in clinical settings. But this is an intermediate experimental phase that is expanding toward the future. The professional dance therapist must have a broad background that is comparable to other disciplines in the hospital setting. She deals in non-verbal communication as a therapeutic tool and uses dance in a knowledgeable way. She can then guide the volunteers and others in using dance on a more superficial level but still in a therapeutic way.

Dance therapy must be under the guidance of a trained leader with definite goals and awareness of the needs of the group. Other dance sessions are useful and are often therapeutic, but a distinction must be made between communication with intention and dance as dance alone.

Movement and Personality

with JARL E. DYRUD

As dance therapist and psychotherapist, we agree that movement and personality are closely interrelated from infancy onward throughout life. As therapists, we are primarily concerned with those people who need help from us, because either their private misery or their public eccentricity has reached such proportions that something has to be done. In either case, we see our task to be one of confronting a problem in the field of expressive behavior. By expressive behavior we mean that which the patient does or does not do to communicate, and his intended or unintended effects upon his environment.

It has long been recognized (at least since Darwin's "The Expression of Emotions in Man and Animals") that human expressive behavior takes many forms beyond the spoken word. The gifted clinician is distinguished from his less gifted colleagues by his ability to understand more than what is said. As Freud said, "he that has eyes to see and ears to hear may convince himself that no mortal can keep a secret. If his lips are silent, he chatters with his fingertips; betrayal oozes out of him at every pore." In spite of this fact, we in the psychiatric field have for years done our teaching, published reporting, and research largely in terms of verbal behavior. It is true that speech behavior is one of the most outstanding characteristics which distinguishes man from other animals. It is also true that the range of verbal expression that man is capable of leads to the possibility of ease in identifying response units and discriminating variations and classes of verbal behavior, which when examined even in terms of ordinary grammatical speech, has a high degree of precision compared to the study of nonverbal behavior.

There is, however, considerable reason to think that our emphasis on the spoken word has defensive qualities as well as the convenience of specificity.

The linguist, Mario Pei, wrote of his fantasy about the origins of language as follows: "In the beginning men had no need for language because they could read each other's minds. When the need arose to conceal what one thought, language developed, along with tacit agreement to ignore the other evidences of expression."

Whether this is historically true or not, we do know that nonverbal behavior can be communication of a very direct form. We also know that it is an expression of emotion rather than of thought, at times in harmony with the spoken word, at other times at variance with it; but at all times requiring a "response" to be understood in contrast to our ability to "track" another person's verbalizations with such responding. When one stays removed from the transaction, as so often happens with verbal communication, understanding of the nonverbal communication will be vague and uncertain. Participation in dialogue which includes the nonverbal elements requires an awareness of our own body responses and those of the other person. Then the vagueness and uncertainty diminish, but the price is greater emotional involvement.

A common denominator of those people designated as mentally ill is failure to sustain participation in just this sort of dialogue. The reasons range from the schizophrenic's intense awareness of and misreading of the signs, to the hysteric's indifference to the subtleties of a relationship.

In the terms of Jacques Lacan, one might say that in all cases the dialogue is interfered with by the patient's reluctance to speak of himself (resistance) and his reluctance to speak to the therapist himself (transference).

The reluctance manifests itself at times in the verbal content. but is most strikingly and reliably observed in distortions of expressive motility. A depressed person, for instance, may show either lassitude or extreme tension, but in either case expressive motility is restricted.

Interestingly enough it has been found in psychopharmacology that the usual initial effect of anti-depressant drugs is apparently not a central effect on affect per se, but a stimulation of the patient to put out more motor behavior. Thus, the agent of change operates directly in the field of expressive movement. An hour of dance exercises preceding a therapeutic hour may have as dramatic an effect on the patient's capacity to express himself as the most potent anti-depressant drug. It has the added feature of organizing the response in a social context which maintains and reinforces such expressive motility. This is not to say that such drugs are unnecessary, but rather than when they are indicated, dance therapy can have an additive effect to channel the new drug-induced propensity to respond rather than leaving its organization and reinforcement to chance.

This organization and reinforcement of expressive movement as an opening move in the development of dialogue has struck us as being more fundamental to dance therapy than the cathartic notion of using it to simply "get out affect." Perhaps the best reasons for our preference for calling this work dance rather than movement therapy is that the word dance emphasizes the expressive aspects of movement. It is true that initially what is important is for some movement to come under the control of the environmental stimulus; the rhythmic beat of the music. Very soon, however, the movement can be related to the therapist's movement also in synchrony with the music, at which point we may say that a truly human relationship is beginning. Often long before the regressed schizophrenic patient comes under the influence of his therapist's spoken word the outlines of dialogue can appear in his hesitant responses to movement with the music and the dance therapist. It may also occur that his earliest organized verbal responses come in the dance therapist's studio. Conversely in the psychotherapy session, gestures or even a change in posture often appear to be the first evidence of remembering an experience which is then followed by the verbalization of it. (G. Mahl)

At this point, we could develop a series of case histories to illustrate this point, but let us assume that it is established. The question is really, "why has the development of psychotherapy proceeded along such verbal and intellectual lines?" Why has our psychology tended to be mental rather than biobehavioral?

The mind-body dichotomy is as old as western civilization, and though it was challenged from time to time by a few offbeat mystics such as Blake or St. Theresa, the major challenge was Freud's insight into mind as metaphor for the experiencing self which was body. The major and popular deviations from Freud were naturally those which reinstated the dichotomy by deemphasizing the irrational and expanding the rational functions of man as mind. The popularity of the various systems of psychoanalytic psychology over the years has seemed to vary directly with the extent to which this exclusion of the body is maintained and people perceived, or conceived of as disembodied ideas.

An unfashionable deviation in the opposite direction was that of Wilhelm Reich. At the time when Freud was being experienced as quite unbearable, Reich not only persisted in emphasizing physical functioning at a conceptual level, but compounded his obnoxiousness by actually involving the body in the psychiatric process. In his book *Character Analysis*, he described how muscle tension is often a resistance blocking the expression of affect. He also described how working directly to release the muscles gave access to a richness of expressive behavior. His work lost much of its professional audience in his later years, yet it has relevance. The expressive behavior which was released by muscle relaxation may very well have been of particular value, because it occurred in a context of beginning dialogue, reestablishing patterns of motility which could then logically extend from motor, to affective and cognitive sequences of increasing adequacy in the dialogue between patient and therapist.

Much of the current literature on child development suggests that this route from motor to affective to cognitive is the normal pattern of growth and development. It is now recognized that the psychomotor development of the child provides the action which is subsequently internalized as thought and feeling. Watching a group of nursery school three year olds, it becomes apparent that their dialogue is in large part one of movement. Verbal behavior is simply less reliable at three. The troubled child moving through a group of children, moves asynchronously with them in crossing the room and simply bumps into more of them than the child who fits into the group and moves with them in an easy and comfortable way. In a subtler way the same is true of adults if we bother to notice.

In summary, we would like to suggest the following train of thought. Expressive behavior in its entirety is the substance of human interaction. The infant's patterns of movement, of action upon and reaction to his environment, gradually become internalized to form his mental and emotional life. In psychiatry there has been a long period of concentration on the verbal aspects of expressive behavior. Now recently, we have come to see more and more interest shown in its nonverbal aspects. Let us hope that this new interest in nonverbal behavior will not be treated like the weather which everyone talks about, but no one does anything about. Counting it or charting it is no substitute for responding to it. Dance therapy is an appropriate way to do something about it. That is, to bring expressive behavior into a more sensitive relationship with the environment. Perhaps to recapitulate the developmental scheme by leading a person deeply alienated from himself and others into dialogue by steps which begin as simply as daring to stretch and daring to move in relation to the dance therapist.

Movement Communication with Children*

The children in this film are in treatment at the Texas Institute of Child Psychiatry of the Texas Children's Hosptial under the direction of Dr. Irvin A. Kraft. They are under psychiatric treatment and at the same time their education is in the care of specially trained school teachers. In addition there is a sports activities program and dance therapy with Mrs. Wynelle Delaney.

Mrs. Delaney is working with this interesting but demanding group of about ten children with much success. These children are overactive and restless, consequently tending to be isolated from their peers and resistant to authority. Hostility is a common theme and probably the one thing they all share. They are more individualistic than one would find among most groups of children. All are above average in intelligence but none can make constructive use of their intelligence.

The film presented for the A.D.T.A. conference was a record of a single session which was under my leadership for the major part of the session while Mrs. Delaney and her assistant aided and then led the latter part of the session.

An interesting aspect of the session was the children's manner of handling an unusual and rather frightening experience with a strange leader in a strange environment. There was complete fragmentation and excitement at the beginning, then developmental work in individual body awareness and then the final expression of awareness of the people around them, relaxation, and acceptance of organization.

At first they were all wild and very active, although each child had different exaggerated reactions to the situation and environment. Since I was a new leader and, so far as they were concerned, had usurped the role of Mrs. Delaney, I at first permitted them to run and investigate the area in which we were working. The children had been instructed to stay within the area of a rug in order to be within camera range and in spite of their excitement, they were able to do this.

* Title of film printed by Sandoz Pharmaceutical Laboratories and shown at this time.

Mary, the only girl in the group, stayed withdrawn for most of the session but even she joined the others before the end. In spite of not being with the group, Mary moved in rhythm to the music so that she gained at least the value of moving/in an organized way.

Philip was very withdrawn and was resistant to joining any group action. At one point he tripped and fell. By empathizing with his feeling of damage to a leg, and manually manipulating his leg into flexing and straightening, it was possible to intrigue him into stretching his body. First he stretched on the floor and then with help did a handstand. This activity interested the other children and some of them also wanted to try the handstand. This was the first beginnings of a group activity. Although the help to Philip had started as giving special attention to him, by being alert to the others as they showed interest, it did not have to remain as that. Soon all of the boys were working at balancing their bodies in the air with varying degrees of success.

Now the boys were aware of themselves and of one another. It was now possible to lead them into the rhythmic action of marching, skipping and jumping in a group. By encouraging one and then another to be the leader, and passing it through the group, another dimension was added. Although Tom and Harry could lead in disrupting a group they were hesitant about leading in an organized activity under guidance. Competition in the jumping remained on a friendly basis.

Harmony was suddenly disrupted by James going off by himself in a pout. This is not uncharacteristic of him.

Mrs. Delaney took over the leadership at this point as we had previously planned in spite of James' disruption. She suggested that they move like some animal. Different animals were chosen readily as this was a familiar game. Two very valuable incidents occurred during this section of the session. Tom chose to use action like that of a chicken. During this he spoke of the chicken of whom he was very fond, who had been killed and about whom he was still grieving.

James was able to come back into the group in the role of a crocodile. As a crocodile, he did not need to acknowledge his return.

Probably the most exciting and gratifying incident was that of Philip. He refused to move like an animal saying that he was a little boy and he wanted to move like a little boy. Since Philip was so frequently withdrawn, this incident was extraordinary. If there had been nothing else that happened, this statement from Philip would have been worth the whole session.

At this point the children moved readily into a customary part of their sessions. They had a reading of a story with the children choosing roles to act out. Today, they chose "The Story of Green Trousers", a fantastic story of trousers that moved by themselves. There is also an opportunity for the children to play reality roles since human children are characters in the story.

The children were quiet and attentive. Many of them lay on the floor on their stomachs, rhythmically kicking their feet as they listened to the reading of the story. When the moment came to act, hands were eagerly raised to show they were ready. There was friendly choosing of roles with everyone involved and a true group feeling. At one point, two boys who are usually loners walked together with arms across shoulders.

The completed film was later viewed by those people involved with the children. It was observed and discussed in sections. The discussion centered on the goals of each section. The reasons for the permissiveness were analyzed as was the over-activity and then the gradual involvement of the children and their acceptance of controls.

My feeling is the session in body action was useful for many of these happenings to occur. Whether a patient shows his tension in overactivity or withdrawal, the first hoped for result is the beginning of relaxation. There are few places where either form of such behavior is an acceptable behavior pattern, but in a dance therapy session these ways of functioning are accepted and worked with from there.

The next section is working with patients in many ways to achieve body awareness. In this session under observation it was achieved by simple acrobatics. When a patient becomes aware of himself, functioning with others will follow. Consequently, the running, jumping and action of role-playing led to interaction with each other. Isolation is cut through and the patient can function for a period of time in a more healthy fashion.

In conclusion, movement communication with children helps to achieve a more relaxed, open child, more aware of self and therefore more able to interact with others.

Music in Dance Therapy

Reprinted courtesy of *Music Journal*, 25 (November, 1967), pp. 25, 67.

In dance, one becomes aware of the close relationship between rhythmic body action and musical rhythms.

Music is frequently divorced from human rhythmic action in our culture. People frequently speak of music that is appropriate for movement; and music which is purely for performing to a listening audience which must remain quiet for true appreciation. This is a logical attitude from the American point of view; but in many cultures the root word for music and dance are the same. It would be inconceivable for people in some parts of the world to remain motionless while music is played or to move together rhythmically except wih the support of music.

One of the places in our culture where this alliance is very obvious is in sessions of rhythmic body action with people who are emotionally disturbed. Even in music appreciation sessions, patients will move quietly in an appropriate way without disturbing others. However, when music is played in a ward, and they feel free to do as they choose, patients will move spontaneously to the music. If they remain quiet, they have usually retreated into their own fantasies are therefore unaware of the environment and a true appreciation of the music being played.

Simple, familiar forms of music are needed for sessions where group interaction is encouraged. It is important that the music used be a base to which they can all relate in individual ways and yet feel a rhythmic action together. It is equally important that an individual be able to relate in different ways to the music, the leader, and members of the group, with his own personal expression of feeling. Each of us has his own responses to the same music. It is the task of the dance therapy leader to permit enough freedom to exist for the patients to move with individual, personal responses, yet remain a cohesive group.

There are always two levels of communication between people when they are together: one is verbal, intellectual communication, and the second is on an emotional, body-action level. While the second level occurs at any time, even though it is often beyond our awareness, music gives support for a group feeling while body action expression is happening in rhythm. The purpose of dance therapy is for communication with one another through this body action with awareness that it is happening.

While many forms of simple music create response and consequent involvement in various people, it is an interesting fact that the waltz music of Johann Strauss is the form that seems to have a universal appeal. Some patients will respond to the lively, clear sound of the polka, others to the syncopated sounds and intensity of Spanish music, still others to the softer rhythmic melodies, but all respond to the Strauss waltz. The tempo is never used by either the dance therapist as leader or the patient group, because the response is to the combination of brightness and the rocking rhythm of the waltz. When this is played, the entire group will become involved in the action without urging.

During a dance therapy session, there will often be patients who cannot tolerate too close a contact with people, who will sit in far corners of the room. However, they will listen to the music and watch the circle of other patients who are moving together in rhythm. They will come out of their preoccupation with their own thoughts and give attention to what is happening.

When the waltz is started, the majority of these patients will move into the group action as though answering a Pied Piper's call, and continue to participate until there is a change of music.

One of the problems of mental patients is confusion about their body image. Therefore, all sessions in rhythmic action are structured not only for non-verbal communication, but also for helping them to have a more definitive awareness of their bodies. This leads to better coördination, more strength in movement, better posture and a consequent feeling of themselves as functioning human beings.

There are many uses of music with rhythmic action in a hospital or clinical setting. Some patients who find it difficult to express emotion verbally are able to express feeling through improvising their own movements to their favorite music. In this case, I do not direct, but empathize by answering in body action in a quiet way from a seat at the side of the room. After they have finished, they will often speak about the feelings they were expressing in movement. Their choice of music ranges from the waltz, again, to Spanish *paso dobles* or more complex music such as a prelude of Bach or ballet music from *Les Sylphides* or *Swan Lake*. When individuals dance in this way they seem to feel a great deal of relief from tension and they relax. Although they are expressing very strong emotion, they never seem to lose control or become upset. Something has been said in movement that they had a strong desire to state in words but could not achieve.

For some patients who are frightened by their feelings of depersonalization, I conduct sessions in which they lie on mats and perform many stretching and limbering exercises. Curiously, although they are working with their muscles, they do not wish to be stimulated by the sound of drum beats, as is the custom in modern dance classes, but again find it most satisfying to move to melodic music, usually the waltz. Again, they often speak freely about their feeling of well-being following the session. It seems to mean enough to them to cause them to be among the people who are most consistent in attending sessions.

When patients feel very debilitated, they will ask to listen to soft melodic music, but very shortly they will be moving rhythmically to it. At first, they will move just their arms and hands, but they soon become involved with their whole bodies and again with a concomitant feeling of well-being. This approach is used most frequently with people who are feeling an overwhelming depression. Many body feelings accompany a feeling of dejection. Patients often are convinced that they have lost an ability to achieve or even to move with their customary efficiency. In this type of session, it is vitally important that the music chosen be whatever the patient enjoys, as well as music that is conducive to helping relaxation. When a patient feels that he can use his body again and can achieve something, however small, some of his fear is dissipated.

One program that has seemed to be of value to the patients at Saint Elizabeth's Hospital has been the use of movement in a candlelight service in the chapel at Christmas. The patients use white robes similar to choir robes. They dance to the Christmas music sung by the chapel choir and use symbolic movement as the Christmas story is read by a chaplain. This use of movement seems to augment the feeling expressed in the

Christmas carols and the Scriptures. The visualization of the words and music keeps the attention of the patient congregation and aids their concentration during the candlelight service. The combining of singing, Scripture reading and movement has become a tradition in the Christmas service at the chapel.

Once a year, the patients write and perform a full-length creative musical drama. They have performed serious drama as well as light, entertaining ones. The choice of music is always their own. One of the most interesting, musically, as well as in the story line and costuming, was the biography of Saint Elizabeth, called *Portrait of Two Crowns*. The twelfth century music, which the music therapist helped them to find, stayed with the audience for a long time in memory. The music chosen was appropriate and beautiful for the gathering of the knights, the folk songs at the German Court and the background for the final tragedy of Saint Elizabeth.

The patients are remarkably sensitive to appropriate and moving music when they are composing ballets. The music must express the same thing that they are saying in dance.

Perhaps the program that received the widest attention and acclaim was the production, *Cry of Humanity*. One ballet was a composition which portrayed the demand for help from Dorothea Lynde Dix by disturbed patients, a moving and powerful interpretation of their own feelings. They used the wailing of music played on a theramin for this. Also in the *Cry of Humanity* was a scene depicting wounded soldiers of the Civil War on the grounds of Saint Elizabeth's Hospital. Their use of *The Battle Hymn of the Republic* was also very sensitive.

In other productions, they have used appropriate music for depicting the implications of a Rorschach card, with the father figure and patient conflicts, the beauty of beginnings of spring, and many other themes.

The combination of music and expressive movement has great significance for the mental patient and dance therapy is a useful tool in the rehabilitation of hospitalized patients, if the music is an integral part of the structure of the goals of all sessions. The integration of music and movement is essential to a program of dance for rehabilitation in the hospital, clinic or special school program.

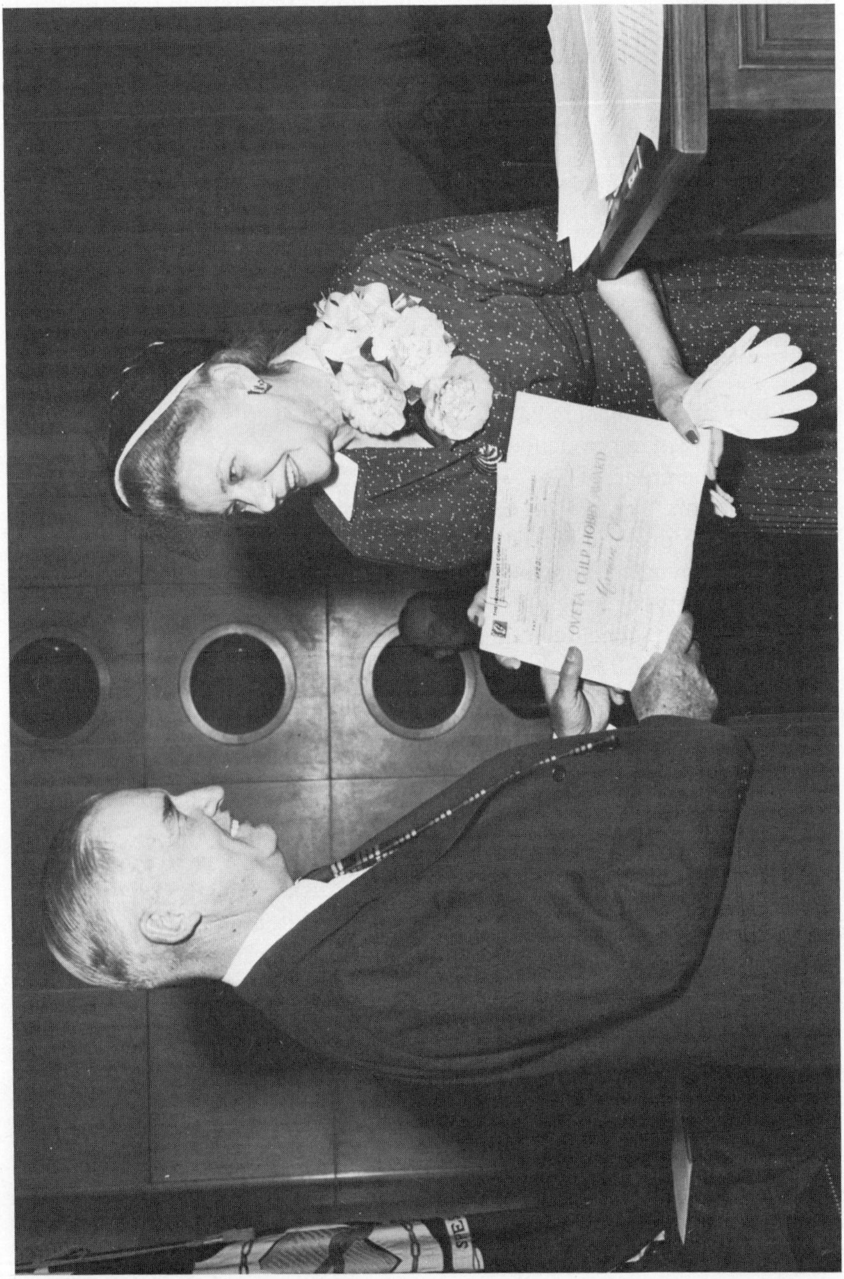

PART III.

Panel Discussions

The Role of the Arts in Therapy

Reprinted courtesy of Northwestern University from *The Northwestern University Reviewing Stand,* 17 (November 11, 1951), pp. 3-9.

with VERNON CLARK, GEORGE M. COHEN and JULIAN PATHMAN.
Moderator: JAMES H. MCBURNEY

Mr. McBurney: I should say, Miss Chace, and gentlemen, that we raise our question today in connection with the meetings of the National Association for Music Therapy now in session here in Chicago. This subject that we are about to discuss very clearly implies that the arts, that is, music, dancing, painting, and the like, are useful in the treatment of certain kinds of disease, at least that they have certain curative powers or qualities. How would you describe the role of the arts in therapy, Dr. Pathman?

'Not a Cure'

Dr. Pathman: I believe there would be general agreement that art in and of itself is not a "cure" for any specific disease entity. We must also consider the various forms of therapy such as the physical, pharmacological, and psychotherapy when we deal in the arts. Art in a general sense may serve as an adjunct or subsidiary to more radical types of therapy, and in this case we must make a distinction between people as people, and people as patients. Now, I imagine that the role of the arts with people would be the role of a prophylaxis. In a more general sense, I would say that art stimulates activity as a creative endeavor, or it may also serve as a diagnostic aid in certain types of illness. Art is a mode of self-expression for certain types of conflicts, both conscious and unconscious, and I think it may also act as a mechanism for the release of emotional tension and possibly in restoring esthetic values in certain individuals. Now, these have different effects with different people and I believe that all these various art forms coud have a definite therapeutic effect.

Mr. McBurney: To make this a bit more specific, Clark, in what kinds of situations or cases can art be used as therapy?

Mr. Clark: Mr. McBurney, I would be at a loss, I think, to call to mind the type of case that could not be helped by some sort of art therapy. It is very widely used with a great variety of cases. For example, it is frequently used with children in certain types of play therapy and of course, we use it extensively with neurotic and psychotic patients we find making up the population of mental hospitals. I, myself, have seen it used and helped use it with patients who have undergone brain surgery. We need something to regain their psychomotor coordination as they recover. In general, we might say it is especially good with patients who for any reason have difficulty expressing themselves verbally in our effort to take them over that relatively mute period when they are unable to bring out their feelings in any other way. I also think we ought to remember that art can be a great help to the normal population, the population at large, in the form of self-help without a therapist but nevertheless as a means of helping them integrate their own feelings.

Use of Dance

Mr. McBurney: We introduced you, Miss Chace, as a dance therapist. How do you use the dance and music in your program?

*Miss Chace:*I use it with the kind of people Mr. Clark was thinking of, particularly those who find it very, very difficult to externalize verbally any of their feelings. I use the dance movement to relate to a patient, and to relate him to other patients forming groups of these people. They are people far out of the picture socially at the moment, who have found other people very difficult to be with. What we do is exaggerate the psychomotor tensions and the action that comes from them into dance movement so there can be a give and take on the non-verbal level and so they can feel comfortable with other people with rhythm.

*Mr. McBurney:*Mr. Cohen, Does this kind of therapy we are discussing have application in your judgment beyond the walls of a mental hospital? It has been suggested that it does.

Mr. Cohen: Here today we are primarily concerned with the role of therapy as a cure, and normal people don't need a cure. Nevertheless, we don't take the "medicine" of art away because there has been a cure effected. It seems to me the expression of the individual through art is essentially healthy, and to give opportunity for expression is a good thing. I might say here I am sort of an apologist for the arts. I am saying art is a good thing as it enables one to give something in the form of his own experience. To be able to project some feeling that he has into a tangible form is essentially a good thing. Just creating a work of art is excellent.

Mr. McBurney: I wonder if it wouldn't be as good an approach as any to get into this subject to talk about Miss Chace's experience with this dance and music therapy. Precisely what are you trying to accomplish with these mental patients?

'At Patients' Level'

Miss Chace: Precisely what I am trying to accomplish is to meet a patient at the level where the patient is at the moment, whether overactive and very quick in changes of mood, feeling very aggressive, or whether the person is very removed. Different techniques are used for both. I do this in moving in with the patient and dancing with the patient who is expressing things in movement that he cannot express and is sometimes very frequently ashamed of. To feel another person is expressing those same things gives him a feeling of being with someone else. On the contrary, someone who is so withdrawn that he is mute and motionless, to feel himself able to move with someone is sometimes a restful thing.

Mr. Clark: Miss Chace, I am interested in what you say about being active. I don't know much about the dance therapy in itself. I would be interested in knowing when a patient comes to you who is very excited, literally dancing on his arrival at the hospital, how do you handle that patient?

Miss Chace: I am told by the people on the ward, the nurses. I am told by the doctor at the head of the service that this person is already expressing in dance movement. Knowing this I can get to the patient quickly and adjust my program to his needs.

Dr. Pathman: That is interesting because I see here a coordination of dance with music in what you are doing. There are certain principles involved, too, which suggest how the arts can be used; for example, if the patient is depressed, you will not play lively music; you attempt to match, as I understand it, the mood of the patient and the mood of the music to get in greater rapport with him.

'Rapport Essential'

Mr. Cohen: It seems then that rapport is essential for communicating—you more or less enter the role of the patient. You establish a kind of music that is in line with the patient's mood. Now, do you feel this is the essential value, that is, communication alone, so that the patient can feel his own attitude is being shared?

Miss Chace: Once a person can share an attitude, then the resocialization process is starting. He can not only tolerate the therapist, but can tolerate other people, and then you can form rhythmic action in a larger group. He begins to feel himself as an entity that is acceptable. In answer to Dr. Pathman's question, when I go into a ward where people are feeling very depressed, I frequently am asked to start the program because I will sit as quietly as the people on the ward until someone suggests that it might be a good idea if I did dance since that was my object in coming.

Mr. McBurney: Do you have evidence that you are getting satisfactory results out of this program?

Miss Chace: I feel so myself because when I am in a ward with very excited people, by the end of the session, people have spilled out their emotions in the action, and are now sitting quietly wanting very quiet music, which is an unusual thing I think on a ward of that sort. When I am on the ward where people are very depressed, I count it a successful session if people are in conversation, movement, and we have had some lively sessions with a lot of laughter.

'Individual to Group'

Mr. Clark: Miss Chace, you have indicated you started off with an individual contact with the patient, and then proceed to a more group expression. Would you say that is typical of dance therapists as a whole, one of the aims descriptive of the process?

Miss Chace: I would think in relating to someone who had difficulty with people, it would be essential.

Mr. McBurney: I suspect that we are talking about a kind of therapy, a kind of program here that is foreign to many of our listeners. I am anxious to get into the basic principles or rationale underlying this whole business. Why do the arts have therapeutic value?

Mr. Cohen: It seems to me this was more or less stated at the outset. The arts being primarily expressive, give the patient an opportunity to externalize some internal state. I think that dancing and music perhaps apply to the socialization of this state, that is, you can share it with others. I think with other arts, poetry or painting or sculpture, you have really a more personal sort of thing. You are externalizing something that is really much more personal. It doesn't take a social form, it is not an established form. I may be wrong about this. Miss Chace, do you feel the dance does have an individual form? In group dancing anyway, it seems to me, you are more or less aligning yourself with a kind of group, whereas with painting you align yourself to yourself.

Miss Chace: Although we are working in groups, there are many people in the session who are unable to be so close to the group that they can conform to the movement of the group. In that case, there is no coercion to cause the person to join the group. Many times we will have someone who prefers to remain individual and express his own feelings and not the group feelings, in which case there is no difference made. Often we have a patient dancing in the middle of the group or around the edges of the group, using the group as a focus and being with them, and yet remaining apart partially.

Mr. McBurney: You are saying over and over again you give these people an opportunity to express themselves. Is it their failure to express themselves that produces their difficulties? Is that the idea, Dr. Pathman?

'Verbalizing Difficulty'

Dr. Pathman: In many cases. Many of the patients and people I have worked with have extreme difficulty in verbalizing. . . .

Mr. McBurney: They can't talk?

Dr. Pathman: They can't talk, won't talk, or are unable to talk for a multitude of reasons. The arts form a wonderful means for allowing them to objectify as it were, some of these inner feelings. There are, of course, various theories of that, sublimation, the escape, the fact we have within us hostile impulses, monsters within us, that we cannot speak or fantasize about; art gives us a media for expression.

Mr. Clark: By doing that though, we can say art therapy is very much like all types of therapy insofar as its aims are concerned. We have used the word "express" over and over, and we have used the word "communicate" which is related to sharing with others. It seems to me we have to think of art as a very typical way of sharing the same aims with other therapists, merely coming in at times when other forms of therapy might not work.

Mr. Cohen: It is interesting to me that we are giving art the reputation of helping us escape and then we are using it in opposition to escape. I should like to mention the thirteen year old girl who defined the arts as "things that you are afraid to say." That was one of the things she added on.

Mr. McBurney: Is that a good definition?

'Afraid to Say'

Mr. Cohen: In this case it is a good definition. These are the things you are afraid to say. However, you don't realize you are saying them. You are putting them into another form. You recognize they are said; they are objectified somewhat; they are outside of you by that time. There is something else that I would like to note here and that is the "monsters" that Dr. Pathman mentioned. I don't think you can describe the particular tensions that are within you as monsters. You can't recognize it as a monster, but drawing or painting or sculpturing can create monsters, monsters that can be a little bit frightening. People don't always like to claim these, but they can come out in these visual terms whereas they can't come out with verbalization.

Mr. Clark: And they can be studied. You used the word "objectify". Anything that has once become real is much less frightening by the fact it becomes real and objectified.

Miss Chace: Often in the dance movements, either with an individual or in the group after having expressed these things with the entire body, the entire self, the patient will then verbalize, "These are my feelings."

Mr. McBurney: I don't wish to be too mundane in the presence of a group of artists, but why wouldn't stamp collecting, sports, or even gardening, have as much therapeutic value as art? You can express yourself, I take it, in a garden or in sports. What do you think about it?

Mr. Cohen: You can express yourself in a garden. We don't judge a person's garden by the fruits of his garden. I mean we *do* judge by the fruits of his garden, but we don't judge it by the way he holds his implements or by his preferences or working habits. Whereas preferences for a technique, preferences for a symbol, preferences for a structure, it seems to me are the essence of art. It is through these preferences we get to understand what a person has done which may lead to diagnosis. And, it is through the presentation of these preferences that the therapy can be worked out.

Passive Participation

Mr. Clark: I don't think we need to exclude stamp collecting, sports or gardening from having a therapeutic role. We can go to the ballet and enjoy our role as spectators even though we do not take part in the dance, and also there are people who collect pictures as well as stamps. We enjoy going to an art gallery and seeing the pictures even though we did not paint them. It is possibly temporary, a more passive form of participating.

Miss Chace: I have often made the mistake when I was first working at the hospital of thinking of a passive participant as one who was not a participant. Eventually one day when he was active I would say, "I am so glad you are with us today"; at which point the remark would be made, "Don't you recognize me? I have been with you for three months."

Mr. Clark: The patient wasn't as passive as she seemed.

Dr. Pathman: The active and passive participants are very interesting. In the passive method you have entirely different goals, whereas in the active type you have I think a greater media for the thinking we spoke about before, the self-expression, the person can actually manipulate and do things in a more active sense.

Mr. Clark: The goals are different, Dr. Pathman?

Dr. Pathman: More limited goals, I would say.

Mr. Clark: Perhaps not more limited. We go to the ballet and art galleries and we see pictures, and on hospital wards whatever we do has immediate results; at least, we hope it will. The effect of seeing a picture may not find any kind of expression for ten years, but I think it becomes an integrated part of the real experience of the person, and therefore has a therapeutic value.

Mr. McBurney: How about these people, Cohen, who can't paint, draw or dance, have no aptitude for these arts you are discussing?

Mr. Cohen: At the outset, there are no such people in our belief.

Mr. McBurney: You haven't met me!

Mr. Cohen: Have you tried it?

Mr. McBurney: No. I think the answer to that should be no.

Mr. Clark: I would question that.

Mr. Cohen: People who do handwriting have a linear gift, and in drawing, people discover they can draw. My role as a teacher isn't to teach them to draw, but let them know that they already can. This is a discovery they have to make, not that I make. The idea of "talent" can keep more people from participating in this therapy than it can bring people into them. People think they have to have a special idea, some special gift for making things, that they have to be a great artist rather than an expressive artist. A similar situation would exist in literature. If people felt that they had to write great novels they would never be able to write expressive letters. We are not looking for great novels or great painting, we are looking for expression.

Dr. Pathman: As therapists, one is not interested in the craftsmanship of the media, but rather in what personal meaning it has for the person and his ability.

Mr. Clark: If I might try to generalize on Mr. Cohen's remarks, the thing he hears from his students, "I can't draw; I can't paint." Therapists call that resistance. We have to recognize that we also as art therapists face a great deal of resistance in many of our patients which has to be worked through. It is unfortunate that the arts have been regarded as something special in our culture; people have been frightened away by the word "talent" by the notion you have to be gifted. The art teacher and the therapist have to be prepared to work through the resistance that we are going to find whether at the social level or whether it is the level of mental disease.

Mr. Cohen: Clark, you are quite right in saying there is resistance to art. I think the artist unfortunately, because of this special gift he is supposed to have, often is regarded as something quite separate. He is regarded as a kind of detached individual who doesn't quite belong to society, but who must be approached with an uncanny attitude. I think there is almost a stigma to wanting to make a drawing or wanting to dance, or wanting to play some music—

Mr. Clark: People want to do it secretly.

Mr. Cohen: They are ashamed. We can always learn from other societies, and in some cultures the artist is the center of the culture. He is the soul-maker; he gives tangible existence to some amorphous idea, an idea of an ancestor, the idea of a God. It is the artist that gives the form. What we are looking for is form given to some intangible feeling, some sensation.

Mr. McBurney: The very fact that this attitude toward art does exist in our culture, unfortunate as it may be in your terms, it seems to me would impose considerable difficulties on the kind of program you are talking about.

Therapy and Society

Mr. Cohen: I am talking here about the broad application of therapy, not only to the individual patient, but to society.

Miss Chace: I very frequently run across the statement of a person who has been working either in painting or in the dance or in music saying, "I had to come to a hospital eventually to do the thing I wanted to do all the time."

Mr. Clark: Quite a horrible thing to have to face as far as our culture is concerned.

Mr. McBurney: To what extent would the effect of this kind of program be, temporary and transient? Do these values that you put on this kind of therapy last? Do they stick with your patients, do you think, Miss Chace?

Miss Chace: Yes, I do very much. I do think it is very wise to have a doctor able to discuss the problem, but with the number of mental patients we have, and the small number of doctors, I think the resocializing is very important. I think once a person can begin to feel himself expressing something, he can tolerate other people, and in that area of resocialization, he can begin to meet society again. I think it does last.

Mr. Clark: And the question is how far will society be willing to go to cooperate with the cure you have given in the mental hospital?

Miss Chace: Unfortunately, that is sadly lacking.

Children and Art

Dr. Pathman: I have something that may be remote here, but I have strong feeling about it and that is the role of our culture. For example, I feel in our curricula in the schools that the children, by working with the various art media, the dance and music and painting, get a feel of the culture, and they can express a great deal about themselves. They can understand therapy themselves and in that way gain an understanding of the culture of other individuals. If we can do that, we are establishing one of the aims of therapy which is in a form of tolerance and of understanding.

Mr. Clark: I am glad you mentioned children, Dr. Pathman. If we watched, we would find that all children without exception, if they have hands, they can draw, but they stop when they are about nine years old. There must be a reason for that. Cohen, I think too, you mentioned knowing other cultures, knowing our own is very important too. If the role of psychotherapy is a kind of self-awareness, understanding of ourselves and our environment, I think even through the passive appreciation of a work of art, we can get some better knowledge of our own culture.

Miss Chace: All children dance too! You mentioned they all paint; they all take activity in all the arts actually, but it is at the age of eight or nine that they stop those too.

Dr. Pathman: There is sort of a stigma attached to artistic types of work in our culture.

Mr. Clark: There is one good theory which gives us some assurance.

When we ask a patient to participate, we are not asking him to do something strange; it is something he has done and enjoyed during his formative years.

'Analyze Experience'

Mr. McBurney: Don't you have to analyze this artistic experience for the patient, at some point in this therapy, translate it into some kind of a constructive interpretation he can understand?

Miss Chace: I don't think it is necessary. When the patient is ready to verbalize and analyze it, he will speak of it often while dancing. He will speak of "this means that I feel so and so." The doctor should handle the actual discussion. I remain as an art therapist.

Mr. McBurney: The doctor should handle it.

Miss Chace: If possible.

Mr. Cohen: There are two roles for therapy. The working out of certain tensions through the release of art on one hand and on the other hand, it can provide a springboard for diagnosis. This, too, is a secondary use of therapy.

Dr. Pathman: I would like to point out the danger of using art to express feeling entirely. Admittedly, catharsis or draining does not solve problems permanently or even remove the causes of emotional conflict. It however prevents intensifying of emotional reaction to a point where they may be detrimental. Alcoholism, for example, might be used by individuals seeking to drain fears and tension, but art would be a more acceptable mode of achieving this catharsis.

Mr. Clark: I would like to go back to your remark, Mr. McBurney, about interpretation. It is nice to be able to interpret at the time or have the doctor do it later, but I think we ought to remember that interpretation involves intellectual understanding. It is a tool of therapy, but not essential with art therapy in bringing about a socialization. I don't think it matters much whether the patient knows that his ability is related to others. The interpretation may or may not happen.

Mr. Cohen: The word "tools" is misleading. It isn't the duty of the therapist to produce the techniques as such. The therapist is a proving ground for this expression. Once the tool becomes more important than the expression, you really have a kind of fine art which is not therapeutic but a demonstration of a technique.

Mr. McBurney: Do you consider this field we are discussing as being ancillary to the primary purpose of art which is essentially an esthetic field?

Mr. Cohen: The notion of esthetics changes a good deal. Respected artists today provide a therapy for society . . .

Announcer: I am sorry to interrupt, but our time is up.

"Our Real Lives Are Lived In Rhythm and Movement."

Reprinted courtesy of *Journal of Health, Physical Education, and Recreation*, 32 (November, 1961), pp. 3-9.

Comments By MARIAN CHACE and WARREN R. JOHNSON
On Movement Therapy for Children and Adults
Selected By BETTIE JANE WOOTEN

An unusual approach to the concept of movement as a force in human lives was presented at the 1961 AAHPER Convention, in the joint meeting held by the Dance Section and the Therapeutics Section of the General Division. The speakers were Marian Chace, dance therapist, St. Elizabeth's Hospital, Washington, D. C., and Warren R. Johnson, professor of health and physical education, University of Maryland. Miss Chace spoke out of her wealth of experience in using dance as a therapeutic measure with adult mental patients. Dr. Johnson's comments elaborated on the film he showed of his work as director of the Children's Physical Developmental Clinic at the University.[1] *The material presented here contrasts and compares the ideas of these two specialists as they relate to specific aspects of the role of movement in therapy. These selections from the convention meeting were made by Bettie Jane Wooten, editor of the National Dance Section.*

The excerpts from Marian Chace's talk are presented within quotation marks; other comments are by Warren R. Johnson.

"The arts, whether painting, music, drama, or dance, are well recognized as being of importance to people as a means for the communication of emotions or ideas that are difficult to translate into verbal forms. The dance, in particular, is perhaps more potent than any other of the art forms. Man lives his life in rhythm and expressive body action, and these are the elements that are involved in dance, whether the primitive religious forms or the social dances of today.

"In our verbal cultures where we rarely grant ourselves the privilege of giving vent to strong emotion, the minute gestures of conversers pass

[1] The Children's Physical Developmental Clinic was organized, under the College of Physical Education, Recreation and Health, in the spring of 1957, in response to a growing need in the Washington, D. C., area for a program which would specialize in improving the physical fitness and/or coordination of subfit children, particularly those generally considered in the special education category. Children referred to the Clinic have symptoms which range from the mild to the very grave—from moderate obesity and more or less faulty movement skills, to brain damage, severe emotional disturbance, and orthopedic disabiltiy.

The functions of the Clinic are to provide (1) an exceptionally valuable training experience for interested students, (2) a laboratory for conducting research concerned with improving child fitness and with studying the effects of improved physical fitness upon the development and educational progress of the children referred to the Clinic, and (3) a unique service to the community.

unobserved or are ignored as though nonexistent. Nevertheless, emotion breaks through the bonds of our strong controls. To quote John Martin in *The Dance*, 'Nature has so constituted us that movement is the medium in which we live our lives. The movements themselves actually have in them the essential nature of the emotional experience even though we have rationally directed them and they do not specifically *mean* anything.'

"The essential aloneness that threatens people generally in our culture is augmented and increased by the distance we are able to maintain. Perhaps it would not seem essential to us to maintain this distance if we dared to express our emotions directly, if we dared to share these with others rather than to hide them and converse in largely emotionless, neat comment. This would not matter so much if there were more frequent agreement between our verbal speech and our inadvertent body actions.

"Our real lives are lived in rhythm and movement, but we rarely share our true feeling. People who are patients in a hospital have exaggerations of the feelings of all people, but no difference in the feelings.

"Certainly, the adult overwhelmed with emotional problems reveals the extreme aspect of this isolation and consequent loneliness. He actually has one asset if the emotions he is revealing are not too overwhelming to others. Conversation is too effortful to participate in when it is concerned with other than his own feelings. These are usually too intense to speak about and consequently he remains alone, expressing his separation from others in body action. He truly is living his life in movement, however much a defeated one.

"Basic dance is perhaps one of the most effective means to cut through this isolation, when the loneliness cannot be expressed in words and the preoccupation with this emotion is too intense to converse about other matters. Even when a lack of initiative prevents a patient from joining a group moving together in rhythm, the observation of such a group in rhythmic action may make a bond which will cut through the distance maintained by the patient. Basic dance is the externalization of those inner feelings which cannot be expressed in rational speech but can only be shared in rhythmic, symbolic action."

It is through this same nonverbal, movement action that children at the clinic are approached. The underlying theory of the personality containing intellectual (verbal) aspects, emotional-social aspects, and physical aspects is assumed.

The usual educational approach is through verbal symbols, that is, through the intellect. But these are children who are emotionally disturbed, who have orthopedic problems, who are mentally retarded, who have emotional-social level problems. Nearly all have some form of retarded development in muscular coordination. They have had the usual related blockages in the learning of academic and social skills.

The child is not in the intellectual-verbal world in which most adult learning occurs. He lives in a world of movement and feeling. In the clinic he is approached in terms of movement; he is approached where he lives.

Nonverbal direction and instruction are used. The first effort is to make friends and see what the child can do without showing up his inadequacies. This must not be another lesson in failure. This must be a lesson to develop confidence in what the body *can* do. the entire personality of this child is resting on the physical base, and this physical base must be strong enough and enduring enough to support and propel the personlity. The entire contact with the environment is through the body. In these cases the body is not under control. By gaining greater control of his body, his basic machine for dealing with life, the child grows in his ability to experience and to learn.

An important difference between the clinic and hospital movement programs in that the mental patients are being helped to return to normalcy, whereas the children are being helped to take developmental steps which are new to them.

The clinician moves with the child, beginning with movement initiated by the child and in which he feels secure. Step by step the movement is broadened or altered so that new experiences are met with confidence and growing control.

"In the hospital a positive quality of aliveness is present in the group of dancers which is in strong contrast to the patients who are sitting listlessly, absorbed in no activity, withdrawn from all others in loneliness. It is exciting to see one of these passively still people rise as though drawn by a magnet and move toward the living group. One must subscribe to the belief that rhythm and a shared emotional experience are important to a feeling of well-being.

Emotions Shown by the Body

"Somewhere in any emotional experience the body enters. People sitting in isolation about the room are expressing this isolation with their posture and the intensity of tension in their musculatures. Whether it is shame, hostility or a general defeat that a patient is experiencing it is reflected in his musculature. Contrariwise, the activity in the group is expressive of sureness, strength, and harmony, and this is translated into an emotion of a positive sort by the people who are either participating or watching. The change in the climate of the area in which the session is taking place can be visibly observed. Bodies that appear weak and inadequate become stronger with vital action. Tension or indifference change to relaxation. Personal commitment to the sharing of an experience takes the place of a commitment to the maintaining of distance from people and a refusal to participate in anything going on which demands the assumption of responsibility.

"The technique for achieving this positive result is through simple rhythms performed in a circular formation. The rhythm must be constantly sustained throughout the session by the leader. Many patients move in ways which are rhythmic by usual standards. Since the patient uses little or no torso action, the movements are generally inadequate and awkward. However, if the leader adapts her movements to those of one of the patients who is involved in what he is doing, others can be led to follow, and a strong support is given to the patient who has initiated the particular movements. The leader then develops the theme of the action using broader movement and involving sets of muscles not used by the patient initiating the dance movement. During the course of the development of the rhythmic sequence, movements initiated by other patients expressing various moods are absorbed into the rapidly changing patterns. While it all seems a spontaneous flow of movement the leader is actually first joining one spontaneous expression in action and then another. From the time that the session begins until it ends, the leader is rarely forced to use her own ideas for the basis of the dance action, provided the ideas expressed in the group are accepted.

"The question is often posed as to whether the physical activity is not the most important part of the dance session. If so, it would be equally effective for the group to participate together in calisthenics. Gymnastic exercise is very valuable and, without question, is an important aid in keeping physically fit, but it does not fulfill the same function that rhythmic action or dance achieves. Dance is not only important as physical exercise but it also involves the emotions through the symbolic movements.

Hostility Expressed Symbolically

"There should be no inference that to describe patients as withdrawn and isolated means they are all passive. I have been describing people with one outward aspect, but the patient is often overactive, restless, and hostile. Talk is almost continuous and scattered. This does not mean any less isolation and loneliness but rather more. Conversation is almost an impossibility as it is too difficult to follow the rapidly changing mood swings. Verbal hostile attacks are more frequent than an attempt to meet the person trying to reach out in conversation. Only frustration can be the result, for this patient is using words to maintain distance, just as another may be using separation in space for this purpose.

"Dance sessions are even more important for this patient than they are for the passive, overtly withdrawn one. The physical activity takes care of his need for exercise and since the majority of his emotional expressions are angry and aggressive it is useful to him to be able to discover that the expression of these hostile feelings can be shared by others, rather than meet only retaliation, usually in the form of a withdrawal from him. There are few instances where his behavior is acceptable or where his actions do not bring retaliation. Whether it is the muscular relaxation through strenuous activity or the shared simple dance actions which can be interpreted as a symbolic expression of destruction there is a comfort in the relaxation that accompanies these rhythmic actions.

"It is difficult to begin a relationship when almost the only way in which a patient can meet another person is with anger, sarcasm, and hostility. In the majority of instances, the only possible reaction of the other person is one that leads to an active quarrel or a rapid withdrawal. This hostility can be met with symbolic battle in dance which will develop into a shared experience that often leads into the beginning of mutual understanding. Answering movement in similar forms dissipates the patient's feeling of apartness, whereas a battle of words can only increase the feeling of separation. Words that are hostile hurt, whereas movements that are symbolically hostile often lead to a warm sharing and a feeling of closeness."

Hostile feelings are often present, and at first often unsuspected, in children playing in the clinic. Some act is necessary, for these hostile feelings must have an outlet. They appear in the activities the child chooses—the punching clown, the trampoline; in the way he attacks the play object—throwing a ball with all his strength; or in his activity relationship with his clinician.

The hostile feeling can be successfully released only if it has a satisfactorily strong, but resilient backboard. Frustration or indifference results from absorption of the overt act, that is, the child needs something that will fight back. Some activities provide a resulting spring or rebound. In the case of hostile physical contact with the clinician, the response needed is a mirror response, matching the feelings and force of the child, not a response of actual anger of the clinician. This response can be the symbol of reaction or the mirrored response of the hostile act, which provides an outlet and yet controls the release of hostility.

The program in the clinic begins with large muscle groups and moves toward use of small muscles. The children tire very easily, and it is necessary to have short periods of rest at frequent intervals. These periods are the time to move naturally toward developing small muscles. The satisfying participation in activity often stimulates the desire to express the essence of the activity, or of the satisfaction, in words—jumping leads to writing about jumping.

"Since ours is a verbal culture we do not wish to deprive ourselves, or anyone, of this important medium of expression. Another phase of the hospital session is the constant flow of conversation. Teaching other people to lead such sessions seems to be one of the most difficult parts of the technique for developing spontaneous involvement and personal commitment of the individual members.

"When the total person becomes a participant in an activity with other individuals it rarely seems important to stay removed from these other people. Changes of mood take place almost visibly and verbal conversation develops.

"As Dr. Joost A. M. Meerloo comments in *The Dance*, 'Man uses many forms of rhythm and dancing to reveal himself. While communicating with others he is invovled in a continuous motoric interaction, moving toward and away from one another. In the unobtrusive dance of conversation, people make minute gestures, they increase their stream of words and sound vibrations inadvertently, or use long silences while their rhythm of breathing changes.' "

Marian Chace uses the term *people* rather than *patients* advisedly. "Dance action is useful in the hospital setting not because the patients are patients but because they are people." And people live their real lives in rhythm and movement.

"The Meaning of Movement: As Human Expression and as an Artistic Communication."

with Jarl E. Dyrud and Jean Erdman

J. Dyrud The theoretical base that I've been interested in is that all of our thoughts and emotions come originally from movement. We start out as infants with action and interacting with our environment. Gradually this action/interaction sequence becomes internalized, becomes a mental life with thoughts and feelings, but it begins in the action sphere and it remains there in much larger part than most people realize. We put a lot of emphasis on words and yet when we interact with other people there is a great deal more expressive behavior that goes on all the time. You begin to realize the importance of expressive behavior and the fact that it doesn't always go with the words. You might say that what ails people is some distortion of their expressive behavior. What we've found at Chestnut Lodge with the deeply regressed schizophrenic patient is that it is very likely that we can recapitulate this developmental sequence that you see in the small child. You reestablish movement first; movement with another person in the dance therapy session. Out of this linking up again in a very elemental way—responding and interacting with the other person's movement, we then see a reorganization of the emotional responses and very often greater organization of the cognitive response.

In recent years I've been working with three year olds in the normal nursery school. Our concern with movement is easy because language isn't a reliable thing with three year olds. What you see most clearly is how reenforcing for them their movement is and also how the distrubed child is clearly out of synchrony with the movement of his group. In walking across a room a disturbed child will simply bump into more youngsters than a happy one. We've been following this up in terms of synchrony or asynchrony of movement and what this means in their lives.

M. Chace: Anyone working with a sick person who has a difficult time with words finds the use of body action and communiction most satisfying. There are responses and true communication going on even though words are not used. The organization and integration that Dr. Dyrud described does occur even if for a short while. Thru this interaction the person becomes aware of himself. He begins to feel his different muscles move in response to action from someone else—not manipulated by someone else—but interacting and it becomes creative because it comes from within the person. This is what dance therapy is about. I've been very impressed down thru the years that I've worked in body action and communication in the split world we all live within. We're so apt to say one thing and *do* something else. The actual doing is the true expression and the words will cover; they may go with it or not but what we do has to be right. Anyone working with patients knows that this is true.

J. Erdman: Hearing this just now makes me feel that these ideas about movement and this activity should go right into every primary school. If every growing child could have the opportunity to develop body awareness and his own creativity out of his body movement, we would have a much better world. We wouldn't have some of the problems that we now have in having to use movement as therapy. If we could develop from the start the full use of one's body, and I don't mean acrobatically but the full spontaneous use of all the possible articulations that we are given at birth, then our whole existence would be on a very much richer level.

Any of you who have taught dance, not as therapy but as dance art know that it is the same thing one does with a beginning dance student. Very often dance students, people who *want* to dance, haven't yet discovered that they have a body. It's funny because they think they are coming to train their bodies, but they don't know they've got one. As Miss Chace and Dr. Dyrud were saying, we move one way and we speak abour something else, or in other words we show our schizophrenia right there. Pardon my inaccurate use of these words. One of the traits of a good actor is that he can find out what sort of movements his character would make which do not correspond to the words he has in his dialogue. If he is a good actor he uses movement to show something about his inner life and lets his words tell you the other part of himself. That makes us rather interesting. Maybe it's good that we have those things that we hide so that they can come out in the movement instead of in the words; maybe that's an enriching thing. I know that actors and dancers actually count on that. Isn't it Rudolph Laban who said that "Man moves to satisfy a need whether it's tangible or intangible", and that's perfectly true. Some of the need he might now want to have known but he moves out of these deep needs. I think a sequel to that thought is that as soon as a man moves, those watching him move know what he wants and even what he needs. It's absolutely self-revealing what you do in movement. Any dance teacher who has a human awareness and not just a knowledge of steps can see a great deal about a human being. Perhaps that's why so many dancers have found dance therapy an exciting area since as a dance teacher one is trying to draw out of the pupil his potentialities and make them real capacities. This automatically implies a human sympathy and a desire to understand more about a person. If the student can be made to come forth more with what he has inside, the dance teacher can guide him to a conscious awareness of his movements so that he can make use of it.

I think we have these two things: human personality and art expression. I think the choreographer, the person who goes into the dance as a way of life and uses this movement language as *his* expression language, is doing soemthing a little bit different from bringing out the possibilities of a human being to move freely and spontaneously. I've always been teaching dance students, in colleges as well as my own studio. What I've found in teaching is that I can always help a young person move to a new stage for himself in his own development as a total person if I can persuade him to deal in creative work or perhaps technical work in areas of movement that he has rejected. For instance I had a student who refused to do any movement that wasn't light and rounded and graceful in the ordinary sense and the idea of doing a movement that was a stamp on the floor, that had a percussive attack or was the opposite of grace, was an anathema. This young girl felt that she had at all times to make herself as attractive as possible and she associated those movements with attractiveness. At that time, she couldn't see that another kind of movement could also be beautiful. When she was finally coaxed into taking on a dance theme that was her own in which she used Bartok's music and another area of movement, that young dancer was able to cope with a much wider range of movement expression. She as a person relaxed in a way too because there was a deeper understanding. Now that's very primitive psychology but it happens all the time that thru the study of dance, people grow. The value of the non-verbal physical approach is so great that we should write manifesto after manifesto after manifesto so that the rest of the world should discover it.

J. Dyrud: I think you have a good point about the fact that non-verbal expression need not always be identical with the verbal, but I think ideally there should be some congruence. You've put your finger on another thing and that was the girl whose expressive range you helped widen. I consider that therapy. Over the years, Marian and I have dealt with people who are extremely restricted in their expressive range. I'm very enthusiastic about dance. For instance, in the case of a depressed patient who is just not putting out much behavior, an hour of dance exercises before the therapeutic hour is tremendously effective in opening up the patient's verbal performance. Another intriguing thing to me are these anti-depressant drugs which people have thought elevated mood. What we find now is that what they actually do is elevate motor behavior, the results of which is a lift in mood. You can do the same thing with dance. Some patients need the drug too but it is impressive that the muscles are so basic in this that you can for a time lift the depression just by getting the patient to stretch and move away from their midline a little bit. I think when you talk about widening the range of expression this does not only apply to deeply psychotic patients but also for the averge citizen who has a lot of muscular defenses against expressive behavior, and who seem tight and flat. A lot of "normal" people are muscularly defended against non-verbal expression and they would get a tremendous lift out of dance therapy when they find themselves opened up and expressing themselves more effectively.

M. Chace: This is very true. I think people are often very startled to discover they can express things with their bodies which they have kept restricted for so long, and that it is not going to be disasterous to be revealing of feelings. I think that a dance teacher does much therapy in this area without calling it therapy. As a matter of fact I started that way myself. I became very interested in why certain people studied dance so consistently when they were not going to be artist-dancers. I wondered what their needs were. This was how I became interested and curious. Certainly we're doing the same thing in bringing movement to people who are very restricted, who are very passive, or who are so over-active and scattered that they can't be organized. Rather than broadening their experience I would say it opens channels to experience. There are some very depressed people who will come consistently for dance action. They are feeling so horrible that they want to begin to feel a little bit better at least on that day and possibly for a longer period. They know that their bodies in responding to movement will cause them to feel better. It's actually a conscious thing. They know this will happen.

J. Erdman: Is it possible for such patients to experience rhythm? Is it something that they do out of themselves or can they actually relate to outside rhythms?

Chace: One could envy the rhythm sense of some of the very sick schizophrenics. I always use outside rhythms. I don't use silent dance at all because they need to relate to the outside. The very thing of being removed from the world will enable them to go back almost to the sense of rhythm that children have. They work with strong simple rhythms, not the complex. The flow of movement and the rhythms are very beautiful.

J. Dyrud: The external rhythm is very important. Even though they "have a sense of rhythm intact" nevertheless what they need is to develop a sequence of behavior. Not that you tell them exactly what to do, but that they begin linking up their own movements into some kind of a sequence in relation to the music first, then to the dance therapist and then to each other. This is not a place for the kind of Merce Cunningham business of just invent in a soundless world. I don't think they would ever get anywhere with it.

J. Erdman: Coming here I was thinking about what the unique thing is about dance that wasn't already in dance therapy. I think it's only the level. Every old medicine man is a healer. He probably also teaches the dances so that the sense of what it is you're healing is the only difference. The artist has to depend on the bodies of the dancers to be well coordinated, beautifully strengthened, richly articulated and very responsive. In other words, the things that get tied up in some one who is ill are untied by the training of the dancer so that the performer has a great deal available to him as a human entity. But that is only the beginning. The art of the dance must create a sense of wholeness and an image of wholeness and a realtionshp in a level that is higher than anything that's experienced on the everyday level. The dancer therefore has to be able to start where an ordinary person leaves off. He must create images through movement of harmonious relationships or of insights into human experience that can be expressed in disharmonious relationships. The main thing is making it a form which is evanescent. It doesn't have any material substance. It is the action which takes place, that creates a form which will feed the spirit of man, which will help him integrate himself with himself and with his environment. The artist has the job of finding images of order which the mind and heart can identify with and contemplate, which are more highly articulated than any individual can think of in his everyday life. The thrill of experience of art is that moment of a new insight into yourself, into the possibilities of ourselves and the possibilities of human relationships. That is the point I would say that man has it within him to supersede himself if he could articulate totally all the possibilities that are there and which each individual person articulates to a certain extent. Everyone of us is different from everyone else because we have selected consciously, unconsciously or in combination certain aspects of possibility of which every human being has the infinite capacity. Yet this is a paradoxical thing. The richness of life is based on diversity and if we were all alike it would be ghastly. If we were all totally articulated in the full circle nobody would have any uniqueness at all. We wouldn't be aware of ourselves or each other because we would all be alike. The limitation which is absolutely essential to an art expression, a deliberate limitation, is the very thing that dance therapy is trying to eliminate, limitations. This is good because it is the only thing that creates form. If you have white light and white sound you have got all the colors put into somethng that becomes pure white color and you have all the vibrations of sound that makes just white sound. You have no shadows to create form. You have no chiaroscuro to give the shading which is the thing that creates the world. We have to appreciate these limitations because it is only through the use of them that the image of totality can be made. The dancer as a human being might be rather neurotic and that is not an excuse for being interesting. You can be interesting in other ways but at least in his vision he knows where he stands. He can point to the image of totality that will be a gift for someone else. It is on that level of responsibility that the dancer as a creative artist is different from the dance teacher or dance therapist who is trying to bring people up to a point of being able to function better as human beings.

J. Dyrud: That is a beautiful statement. I am glad you brought in the neurotic because I was thinking of Nijinski who danced very well and died schizophrenic. I would not say that what Marian and I are advocating is that we get a standardized communicating human. Each individual can develop his own unique capacities. The distinction is that in dance therapy you are not trying to create artists. You are trying to create communicators and are trying to help people engage in more meaningful dialogue. One of the unnecessary tragedies that happens with some dancers is that they become privately tied up with their own bodies and very poor communicators with their fellow humans. I don't think this adds to the dance. We were discussing whether in fact the best artist is not the one who has the best rapport with the audience. You see some dancers who you feel are dancing with and for themselves alone and this does shut you out, except in so far as you can identify with it, which is quite different from communicating with it.

M. Chace: They permit you to identify with it which is a very lonely state and a very empty one, whereas other artists do communicate. They have an idea which they wish to communicate. I don't mean they come out and feed the audience but communicate ideas. They are the most vital dancers. I don't feel that art forms are completely left out in doing dance therapy with the patient. They reach out for expressions that are beyond themselves often times. The difference is that the artist has an intentional idea to communicate whereas the patient is expressing something from within himself which is not his purposeful intention to communicate. It reaches out and does touch people but it is not with that intention. This is one of the areas where there is a difference between the artist and a patient in a dance therapy session.

J. Erdman: It seems to me that communication takes place when the expression is vivid and complete and total. Why should one be intentional about communication?

M. Chace: If you get up on the stage you intend for people to understand what you are saying. You'll find many times that schizophrenics have no intention of your following them. As a matter of fact it is rather disturbing if you do.

J. Erdman: In other words they don't want to communicate but rather stay within themselves. Does that correspond in your thought to what you were saying about some dancers who don't communicate? They are acting like patients in a sense?

M. Chace: Yes, they are depersonalizing their work. They mean to say what they say but they don't mean to share or project or communicate. That is depersonalizing it.

J. Erdman: I always think of things in reciprocal rhythms. It seems to me that part of a human being is his openness and sympathy, taking in things and being aware of someone else. Then there is nothing of himself. He is taking something in. The other part of him is his need to express or need to create and he isn't thinking of anybody. He is getting this thing out and the act of actually having to communicate is not necessary.

J. Dyrud: Let's begin with the premise that when you engage in conversation with a person you may be quite remote from it and you're simply dealing with it at a cerebral level. If you respond at a non-verbal level the only way you read the other person's nonverbal behavior is by your response which is quite a different order of things from tracking his words with your mind. The patients we see at the beginning do not in this sense respond because they can not risk the emotional involvement that comes with responding and reading another person. Dance work is a very innocuous way in which you can begin the process of reading and responding to the music and to the other person's movement. It leads into more communicative responding over time. The artist who is, and I like the way you put it, presenting a creation, a beautiful idea, may not have anything to do with responding with another human being at all. It may be between himself, the music and the idea. That is why it is quite possible for a dancer to be quite withdrawn socially and still be very expressive on the stage. What puzzles me in this discussion is the dancer who goes through these preparatory steps of which you are speaking and yet doesn't come up with both the artist's creation and a human being.

J. Erdman: I think they do come up with being a human being. You are the guys that have said they are not. I think dancers are humans, though as a matter of fact dancers we all know have been labeled, and they probably deserve it, auto-erotic narcissists. Maybe it is because they have to work on their own body so much and stand in front of a mirror. Some get past that but not all. People, at least in creative dance, who are interested in choreography and in new forms of dance tend to be philosophically inclined. Actors are quite the opposite. They are always looking at other people trying to catch the spirit of someone else so they can recreate it on the stage. The dancer can find the answer to life in a philosophical way within this one body moving beautifully in front of the mirror. The movement is sensed as totally kinesthetic in all the elements of motion, of time and dynamics and the whole thing becomes a very total world. I meant to speak on behalf of those dancers that you call cold, non-communicative people. The dance artist who has really gone to work through this narrow path of working on his own body to a point where he can do things that other people can not do, not just to show off but for the purpose of being expressive about human life, is to proffer what people used to call in the old times icons. Of course he can get all fouled up with figuring himself as one of those gods, but he presents in his dance work that kind of image. It doesn't have to communicate on the level that we generally do from person to person. It can be such an image that it catches everyone in it. I don't think that the only way to judge the depth of humanity of an artist's work or the artist as a person is his communication.

J. Dyrud: I would agree. I am sorry that Nijinski had to die in a mental hospital just as I am sorry that Vincent Van Gogh died in one. It is nothing against their art but as a clinician I think it is a shame that both sides don't develop.

J. Erdman: I think they do in some people and they don't in others. What I would resist is to classify artists and particularly dancers as predominately that kind because there are plenty of people who aren't in the arts at all who are like that. It is not necessarily the dance that makes them that way.

J. Dyrud: However, I would think that in teaching dance to people who are going to go on and become great creative artists in the dance, it seems within reason that we could knowingly help them develop some communicative skills along the way to avoid some of the hazards.

J. Erdman: I don't think that it is so hazardous. I guess that I am for the madness that it all is. Take the statement that is made by the ballet. You can't say that Nijinski makes a statement or Nureyev makes a statement. The ballet is making the statement. The art of the ballet is an anonymous art and the personalities performing within it bring a certain little nuance to it by their unique personalities. But what is being said through the art is something that comes about because of the choices that were made within the realm of possible areas of movement that belong to the ballet technique. When you look at Martha Graham you see something you can say is her statement because she chose everyone of the limitations that she decided characterize the quality of movement and the technique and so on and left all the others out. The individual who chooses to make similar choices we can identify as a Martha Graham type. Anyone who repeats that movement has lost its original expressivity but for Martha Graham's art she found all the choices that were necessary to create *her* image of totality, her image of man's relationship to the universe and it has a certain character. It is from a certain standpoint and expresses truth from a certain vantage point. If the person Martha Graham had not the particular limitations within her character and personality that made her choices so as to be her opus of self-revelation, we wouldn't have had the art. To help any individual getting started as a creative artist to help him to be better adjusted and more understanding of others and himself, might deprive him of the need he would have for his art expression. This in a sense is like publicly working out your neurosis but on the way you are giving people gifts of your experience, of your own insight if you are a real artist. That might not be the art you like but that is because your own personal needs were not the same. In a classical art or an anonymous art like the ballet, it is sayng something very specific about man's relation to the universe. If you don't have a limitation and a point of view, you can't make a statement.

J. Dyrud: I was not attacking creative dance. I was thinking dancers I have known have been forced to live a very rigorous monastic existence for many years and they may have some sort of occupational hazards. The restriction of behavior that goes into becoming a prima ballerina are tremendous and this may well be very restrictive of her social communicative functioning. In that sense it is a hazard.

Question: I am not in dance therapy and I know very little about it but it seems to me that what you are talking about is similar and that is that you are both using movement to help people to find themselves. The dancer, when he starts moving is finding himself and then as he performs he is helping the people in the audience to experience ideas and feelings and as a result to help them find themselves. You can compare the dancer in that capability with the therapist who is also trying to help other people find themselves but not vicariously by watching, but by experiencing. This is why I think we got off by comparing the dancer and the patient. We should be comparing the performer-dancer with the therapist who are kind of working in the same way trying to help other people find themselves through movement. Is this what you are getting at?

M. Chace: I don't know that comparing it to the therapist is the thing because the patient who is dancing and the dancer are the two different people attempting to solve an idea with movement and with rhythmic movement. The therapist is on the side lines enabling the person to achieve this.

Question: It seems to be nowadays that the training of many young dancers almost mitigates against their expressing themselves through the dance. I find through workshops with dancers that they are infinitely less expressive than the patients I work with. They have to break through to find themselves in movement because they put out a little of Martha Graham here and a little of Hanya Holm there and they don't know where they are at in terms of their own bodily expression. You have to dig very deep sometimes and maybe this is something with which you have to deal.

J. Erdman: That is very true, When young dance students identify with a certain kind of dance training and then try to use it, they don't know that they are not assimilating it to themselves and recreating it. They don't know what they are missing because they have been taught it and think that is what dance is about. If the art of contemporary American dancers, in creative dance rather than as traditional art, is personally based, it absolutely belongs to that individual and anybody who repeats it is going to be that much less convincing in his art and in his person. He will be shutting something off from himself. It's only in the traditions of folk dance which express a whole culture or a whole people at a certain time that the individual human being is not frustrated in his relationship to repeating movement. The necessity that is very apparent is to find ways for dancers to keep in touch with themselves while learning the skills that are given them and learning to interpret the work of an individual choreographer. For instance, Hanya Holm pedagogy always included improvisation and always included work for each dancer to discover his own style for himself. It is certainly the attitude of Alwin Nikolais' group. The only thing is that now Nikolais' place is so efficient that people don't know that they are not discovering themselves because they have learned so many devices for creative work. The devices become the thing that replace their own individual search.

Question: I am curious as to the differences between dance therapy and movement therapy or is it just terminology?

M. Chace: It is a terminology but there are various forms of movement theapy. I think dance therapy specifically includes rhythms.

Question: I am coming to the defense of the modern artist whether he be a dancer, musician or painter because if we go back in history many of the artists that we readily accept and understand today were unacceptable in their early stages, like Picasso, Schonberg and others. Isn't it then true that society and the people have to be developed into an understanding of communication whether it be in painting, music or the dance?

J. Erdman: Now that is the point that I was making. I wasn't saying that people become unneurotic by their work. They can possibly work through to that. What they are doing is creating images of order from a certain standpoint which are self-revelatory, are something to experience as a new image of order and they wouldn't be understood right away. The modern artist in our civilization, in Europe and America, is a celebration of our regard for diversity and the individual uniqueness of human beings. If your work as therapist is to help people to become themselves you are helping people to become different from each other, not all alike. The artist is simply standing on that premise and trying, out of a vision hopefully large enough, to present something to look forward to, to expand one's own sense of the balance or imbalance of things. It's a self-standing image that is to be experienced as a new experience. That's what a modern artist is as opposed to a traditional one and that is what an individually signed piece of work is as opposed to an anonymous one.

Question: Haven't you found that there are times in working with the ill person when the ill person is really more honest in his distracted communication or lack of communication than the well person?

M. Chace: I don't find them having lack of communication. He has tremendous communication on the body action level which is where I work. One interesting thing about the very ill person is that he has no grays to his concept. He is all black or all white. I think that he is more honest and it is very refreshing.

Question: Is it just a question of how it fits in with our civilized society?

J. Dyrud: I would be a little leary of that. This is the notion of the brilliant insightfulness of the very disturbed patient and it is not so.

M. Chace: But he demands honesty.

J. Dyrud: He demands it from you. That is entirely different. One of the reasons that the disturbed patient is disturbed is his distorted view of what's what. There is not much point in talking about his honesty because he may say honestly a number of very strange, inappropriate and irrelevant things.

Question: I would like to go back to the question of whether dancers are able to work out their neurosis through their art. We talked about the therapeutic effects of the dance in education. We all know that everybody who has danced has received some form of therapy but what we are doing in our work is seeing that we are psychologically directed towards a certain goal, achieving a desire to step from one state to another. This is where therapy differs from plain dance education. The art itself is therapeutic but because it is not directed, dancers can be neurotic. One might also ask had Nijinski not danced would he have made it to the hospital much earlier?

Question: There was a statement made that limitation was something that dance therapy was trying to do away with and that hasn't been my experience. The rhythm is in patients, and this is the greatest aid that we have to help set limits. Stronger limitation in the setting is what they are in need of so desperately. Rhythm is the greatest tool that we have to achieve this and those limits then can also help bring about more appropriate behavior.

J. Erdman: People who are psychotic have had their flexibility as human beings limited to such an extent that they need to have limitations done away with so that they can function. That is the kind of limitation of which I was speaking. What you are saying is that people need a sense of order and form in order to function well. So does an artist if he is going to make a statement. He has to have a choice of elements. He can't just use every old thing or otherwise there's confusion. You are trying to work with hman beings who are in such trouble that they cannot function. I remember hearing Irmgard Bartenieff saying that she was working with patients who were greatly disturbed. The first thing that disappeared in their movements were the complete rotation of a joint. In other words they tended not to use the full rotation but only to make a limited use of it. There is a kind of flexibility that is natural and that would be limited by the illness. This kind of limitation is what dance therapy eliminates. I was so interested to hear how important rhythm is for you. Dance doesn't exist except through limitations that have been chosen in time, space, energy and flow if you want to go all the way to Laban. So the *use* of dance is important, the use of carefully understood elements of limitation can help to bring people out of their problems and give them the full use of their arms. You see where the two limitations got mixed up.

J. Dyrud: This may be carrying it too far along but I would like to extend that comment. The reason that the rhythm is so important is that the very disturbed patient's behavior is not closely tuned to the environment and the therapist is largely ignored. About the first vehicle for sensitizing him to responding to his environment is the beat. It may well be that music is too threatening. You may simply have to use a tom-tom or something. What you will find is that if you start with some very elementary rhythm, you are trying to hook his behavior into something that you are doing and then you can build on that. You begin with a person who is not hooked in at all to anything you are doing and it organizes his behavior.

J. Erdman: Rhythm is so important in my thinking about expressivity that it seems to me that it is the essential element to expression entirely in the use of every art. It is the one thing that unites all the arts. When you speak about rhythm dynamically, the different kinds of rhythms, it is in the rhythm that the core of expressivity resides. It is the thing that gives form. The Hindus have a marvelous idea. I am sure you must experience this in your work. Each one of us is made up of a huge sum of varying vibrations which are rhythms. Let's take Dr. Dyrud because he is here. If we could figure out every one of the vibrations that are right for him, if we could find every one of them and see each rhythm in its proportion and recreate those vibrations in rhythm, sound them out, we could put another one of him right over here. He would come into being because we are made up of energy in a rhythm. The Hindus of course are a magical type people, at least in their books. I believe it can happen, but of course you can never get that last little vibration that would clue it into the whole and make it a unit. But when we respond to each other in movement and sensory ways, non-verbal, physical ways, it certainly has to do with our rapport of rhythms. When dancers learn to improvise together they learn to trust one anothers rhythms and relate in those terms. I think it is fascinating to hear this is used as one of the main tools of dance therapy.

PART IV

Unpublished Papers

Marian's unpublished works probably are equal to the size of what is contained in this volume. They were particularly hard to locate. In addition, there are several tapes that need to be transcribed and made available. A limited selection of this material is included here. Perhaps it will spur others to locate and assemble this material.

A Psychological Study as Applied to Dance

The arts are used today in the institutional setting with increasing enthusiasm. However, the attitudes of the medical therapists toward them vary a great deal depending upon the institutions with which they are associated and their own preconceived attitudes toward art and artists as well as their direct contact with one of the arts. This is not all to say that their attitudes are always on the negative side nor even in the majority of cases. Art is often spelled with capital letters and imbued with some mystery which is frequently thought to be beyond comprehension by the average man.

The person who is working seriously in the arts, however, sees whatever mode of expression he is using as nonverbal communication. This is true whether he is painting on canvas, composing or performing musical compositions or participating in drama or the dance in the theatre. No work of art is of any value unless there is a direct communication from the artist to his audience. This does not beg the issue that this audience is more often a small rather than a large one. Nor am I saying that the artist does not often speak in abstract or emotional terms that are sometimes obscure to a great many people.

A lack of understanding of the fact that there must be a direct communication in an art form often results in an over-enthusiastic acceptance of the artist as a therapist in a medical setting. The idea that art forms are intelligible to artists, but are perhaps too complex to be readily understood by others is a fallacy. Only if the artist was sufficiently clear in his concepts for people outside of the hospital, is his work within the hospital of value. Only when the teacher himself has had sufficient satisfaction through his ability to communicate feelings and ideas can he become interested in the communication of others. Patients need to use some art form as a satisfactory means of communication for it to be a therapeutic tool for them. They should never be led into fulfilling the needs of the therapist who is using one of the arts as a tool for his own satisfaction. This must be more clearly understood before the mystery can vanish and a technique for the use of art in a therapeutic setting be developed.

Sometimes the use of an art form is either valueless or actually harmful to a patient. Occasionally, it can even be used to augment his isolation and become a means of strengthening his fantasies. Unless people generally begin to understand that art is valuable to patients only as it gives them a means for communicating feelings in a direct way can there be an understanding of what happens when art is used.

What, then, can be done about this situation? Study of what goes on between people in the setting of an art session is the only conceivable answer, and yet no field of science has been able to establish tools for measuring the processes involved in empathy and affect. Events of varying sorts occur which lead us to believe that empathy has been established between people. People change in their outward and observable behavior patterns in such a way that it can be believed that their response to given social situations has altered. However, exactly what happened or what combination of circumstances was responsible for what happened remain in the area of intangibles. Nevertheless, some evaluation must be made of when and why sessions are helpful and when they are harmful. This must be done especially in the area of music and the dance. Otherwise much that is helpful will be understood only vaguely and much that is harmful will go unnoticed.

Communication through an art form is based entirely on empathy and affect. What then is it possible to measure in such sessions with our present tools? Great conflict rises in a person such as myself, who is working in the dance who recognizes the need for validation of what goes on in dance sessions and yet acknowledges the impossibility of measuring the elements which seem to be the most important ones. It is not enough to feel that communication does exist between patients who are moving together. It is insufficient to feel that as a patient experiences the creative outlet of dance, either alone or with others, that he gains in self confidence, establishes relationships with others, and becomes more of an entity who is aware of himself and therefore has gained in the possibility of functioning more adequately. It is important that the factors contributing to this be measured. Only in this way may such sessions be better understood or distorted, in an attempt to understand. It is not enough to believe that communication on a nonverbal level goes on and that empathy is established among members of a group.

One frustration for the artist leader in an attempt to study this process is that he can be only a participating member of the group to be studied. The very nature of his work, that of nonverbal communication, necessitates an intense personal involvement, which immediately eliminates him as a valid objective evaluator. If he steps out of his role, there is no session to evaluate; his direct communication with another person is lost.

During the past summer I engaged in such a study with a student in the Psychology Department at Saint Elizabeths Hospital for his Master's thesis. I am aware that as a leader of the group, and therefore the activating tool for achieving changes in the group members which may possibly be measured, I offered a problem of many variables. In setting up the study, therefore, we accepted the fact that I would be a continuing variable as the leader.

Another difficulty lay in the fact that dance therapy as conducted at Saint Elizabeths Hospital does not follow a rigid routine in the dance sessions. The sessions begin with simple relaxing exercises for stretching the large muslces and bending the joints to the accompaniment of waltz music. Following this, however, sessions are governed by immediate response to situations developing in the group. It was decided that since we were studying possible changes which might take place in the patients during the course of these particular dance sessions, it would be necessary for me to conduct them as usual. Certainly this was fortunate for me, as I would have been very awkward in any other manner of functioning, and I would have felt that the dance sessions must remain on a spontaneous level in the fallacy of attempting to rate dance actively on a standardized scale based on stereotyped movements. The scales can be so devised, however, that the sessions may be on a spontaneous level and can increase in complexity with the growing alertness of the patients and consequently this danger can be avoided.

I accepted the fact that the important areas for study, those which deal with empathy and affect, are impossible to evaluate with the present tools for measurement. I understand the reasons for a base from which to start and scales showing progress from this base, which can be tabulated for objective evaluation. But also, since empathy, affect, and the development of interpersonal relationships are the stuff of which dance sessions are made, how could anything meaningful be measured? Why attempt to measure anything at all? Since I feel that somehow we must try to validate what happens, I was willing to try. I was interested in whether, as an end product, some of these intangible things could be measured in terms of present day methods. Perhaps somewhere some fact of clinical observation might be related to an objective study.

In order to circumvent as much as possible the question as to whether changes in the patients were largely due to sessions of rhythmic action in a group, we were limited in our choice of patients to those who were very passive and who consequently were involved in no other program of any sort.

Our group of patients, both those in the control group and those in the dance group, were chosen first for the fact that they were schizophrenic, second, that they were not participating in any activity or receiving any form of therapy and, third, that they lay within the age range of 20 to 40 years. The combination of these criteria limited us to patients who had been hospitalized from five to twenty years.

The evaluation of change in patients within the group is by means of the projective drawing test given by the psychology student and evaluated under the guidance of her supervisor. The number of patients in such a passive group who could make even a recognizable attempt to draw was less than the number originally selected for the study, and we started to work with 17 men and 14 women in the dance group and an equal number in the control group, who were matched as to Goodenough Score, length of hospitalization, age, and those taking tranquillizing drugs. The majority of the patients were either not verbalizing at all or occasionally spoke only a word or two with people with whom they had been closely associated for a long period of time.

Obviously, with such a group, minor changes on a social level might conceivably happen, although it was equally conceivable that changes of a nature deep enough to be evaluated objectively might not be possible. We know that these changes on the social level, while important to individual patients, would probably be in the area of intangibles and consequently immeasurable happenings. All communication at first would have to be on a nonverbal level. We hoped that empathy would develop between the leader and individual patients and that they would begin to develop evidence of more energy, longer periods of concentration, brightening of the eyes, and occasional smiles instead of expressionless faces, self respect shown by helping with furniture, more pride in appearance, moments of initiative rather than an outward evidence of dependency and the ability to give and accept expressions of friendship and hostility. All of these things which develop in a series of dance sessions and are the important happenings in the rehabilitation of a patient would have to be ignored. There are not tools for the evaluation of such things. This is where the leader of such a group feels intense frustration. All of the gauges by which the dance leader judges whether these sessions are of value to the individual patients must be discarded. It is a difficult bridge for the person working in the arts to know and accept the fact that although working within a structured study, for the purpose of evaluating the help that dance might be to a patient, those things which relate specifically to communication on a nonverbal level in dance form are the things to be discarded in the study, even though they are of major importance to the leader, and apparently give satisfaction to a patient. For instance, in the men's group the leader frequently used aggressive action with both arms and legs. At first, none of the men were able to drive forward with their fists. It was apparently a frightening gesture. However, eventually, they could use their arms in strong movements toward the leader. The degree of force that a patient used could be measured, but not the apparent satisfaction he exhibited in doing the gesture.

Although the possible changes in the projective drawing tests were the particular focus of this study, we were also interested in a possible correlation between changes in the activity, increase in freedom of movement, development in initiative, and growing awareness of the group with the possible chance of no change in the projective drawing test at the end of twenty-three sessions. This, of course, was my principal interest. I knew that these changes would occur, but I had no way of knowing whether these changes would show on any psychological tests.

In structuring the way in which to make evaluations of the activity of individual patients and the group as a whole, we finally decided to use two objective observers who would check at five minute intervals the movements made by the patients during the session. They were to note any sort of movement with any degree of force which was in rhythm with the music or related to the activity of the group. In order to complete the picture, however inadequately, and only because my interest lay in this direction, I worked out a five point scale which would show observable development of group awareness, initiative in activity which is appropriate to the group action, leadership in the group, and length of concentration of the activity. While all of this is important to the individual patients, the evaluation of such things would necessarily be judged subjectively by the leader and consequently would not be scientifically valid.

As the patients grew accustomed to the sessions and became more at ease with the leader and the other members of the group, the check on movement at five minute intervals became almost meaningless. Nearly all the patients were in action at all times. By the seventh session we became aware that we must add another scale which would give, but again only inadequately, the degree of freedom and force of the movements of the movements of the patients.

Movement, as such, is even more complicated than the emotional experience out of it, or the relationship established through it. In accurately describing a rhythmic action in terms of a scale one must take into consideration rhythm, coordination, partial or total body involvement, energy, force, direction, relaxation, tension, and freedom. In attempting to make a scale for all this we devised one which ranged from constricted action of the limbs close to the body to full coordinated movement originating from the body as a center and extending beyond the extremities into awareness of the space beyond the patient. This would inevitably show the amount of force exerted in a movement. Movement close to the body without trunk involvement is lacking in energy, and that with full movement can be made only with directed force. We are uncertain, however, as to whether people who are not dancers or athletes are aware of this. In addition, we were unable to include the emotional quality of the movement as, again, there is no tool for measurement. Perhaps through our scales of frequency of movement, degree of force of movement, tabulated by the objective observers, together with my subjective scale of a patient's involvement with the group movement, which also indicated involvement with the group members, we will be able to give an adequate picture of what went on in the group during the 23 sessions. This will remain to be seen.

My frustration still lies, however, in the fact that the really important things happening to the patients are of necessity being ignored in the study. The changing attitudes of the patients which mean the beginnings of steps toward a desire to function in more satisfying ways are still not measurable even though these steps are observable through the changes in behavior patterns. Smiles, the first hearty laugh by a patient who does not speak, tenderness expressed toward the leader, development of verbal speech, buoyant steps instead of dragging shuffles, people able to take leadership, are not daily happenings. These things are obviously the result of the dance action in the group session but they cannot be measured by present methods. All of the measurable things could happen in any activity in a group setting. Beyond this lies the observable pleasure and relaxation from moving in a satisfactory way with music rhythms and listening to tonal sounds with people who are becoming familiar. This is the essential quality of a dance session, and is totally outside the limits of objective evaluation.

However, one learns that to be the leader of a group involved in such a study is by no means a completely frustrating experience, but rather a rewarding one in many ways. The need to rate activity on an established scale does not block spontaneity in an activity but rather helps one to be more ready to meet the needs that are being shown by the members of the group. In other words, one finds certain aspects of awareness sharpened and made more acute.

In spite of the lack of ability to measure the happenings that are important to individual patients and the group as a whole, as it begins to form one becomes even more aware of the complexities of these happenings and the need for much further study in the area of nonverbal communication. When one works in the area of dance with either nonverbalizing or inadequate verbalizing people one becomes increasingly aware of the richness of expression through body action. Translating an evaluation of nonverbal communication into a scale which is understandable to others who have not had the particular emotional experience, one is increasingly aware of the complexity of this experience, in a very poignant way. When no specific evaluation is necessary, one has a tendency only to feel about it and rarely to attempt to express it with clarity in words.

Since one functions in dance sessions almost completely on a nonverbal level, much may be missed in the very acceptance of this form of communication. The awareness of interaction with one or more people in dance is a comparatively simple matter when it is left in the feeling area. Provided the leader does not attempt to translate this feeling into words, he feels what has been going on and can answer spontaneously and verbally what has been said only in movement by the patient. There are so many nuances and complexities in this experience that one would need a scale of unwieldy length to describe accurately even one small incident. To be specific about an experience, however, can be done only with words. One becomes far more alert to comparatively exact meaning, and consequently more precise in answering what is being expressed on an emotional level and with no loss in empathy or emotional awareness.

This study had not been completed in time to report in this paper as to whether there was any correlation between what actually went on with the patient during the sessions on a social level and the second projectie drawing test, or whether there was an appreciable difference between the tests of the dance group and those of the control group. Nevertheless, as with an experience in any art form, much went on to create a more satisfactory experience for individual patients.

It is unfortunate that in a study such as this, one must limit that which is being evaluated to a point where no picture of the reality of the experience is possible; but rather a distorted view. Few experiences involve the total person as completely as that of dance action: the body, the emotions and the mind. Moving with other people in a similar rhythm often helps relationships to form within the group. Yet our scales can give only the most partial and superficial evaluation of all this. Part of the difficulty lies in the use of verbally oriented scales for a nonverbal medium, and even the final test, while nonverbal, will evaluate only a small fraction of the total experience.

Dance and other forms as used in a therapeutic situation must be evaluated. It should be possible to know when the use of it is beneficial or when it is harmful. Standards of leadership for such sessions should also be developed. However, until a test is devised which does not require translation into verbal forms for the evaluation of emotion experience, we will be at almost a total loss in attempting studies involving nonverbal communication. When some one thinks through a totally new nonverbal test which will be neither an adaptation, a restriction, nor an augmentation of one suited to other media that we continue to try to understand that process that leads toward resocialization in this complex field of expression and the related nonverbal communication.

However, as new means of validation are sought in the area of nonverbal communication and creative expression, let us keep in mind that there is little uncertainty in the day-to-day working situation, but rather in inadequate means to validate scientifically what is being felt. It may be that it will continue to remain intangible. It will certainly do so while we remain bound to present limitations of scientific methodology as applied to the intangibles of human interaction in nonverbal areas.

The Arts and Mental Illness

A major problem in working with patients in any of the arts is the necessity to keep a proper perspective on the area in which encouragement can be useful and the area in which it can be defeating. This is particularly true where the patient has an unmistakable talent or skill. When I speak of unmistakable talent I am speaking in terms of the hospital population. A patient who seems remarkable here would rarely stand out in the field of his interest outside of the hospital. So many of the people with whom we work at the hospital show little ability to carry through on even simple projects that it is very important to many of the staff to discover someone who is different from the average. There is a centering of interest on the patient's skill and the use of this talent often is seen as a solution for future planning.

The patient himself enters into this solution as, for the first time, he is suddenly recognized as being different, glamorous, and able to be outstanding with little or no effort on his own part.

This well-meaning attitude on the part of some members of the staff who have no familiarity with the qualifications needed by the artist for earning enough money to pay for rent, food, and the bare essentials of living creates a serious problem for those who are using the arts as tools as an outlet for the patients while they are hospitalized.

I am presenting the following problems at the beginning of this presentation rather than at the end, as I see them as relating to many patients rather than relating to a specific case.

1. How can communication be strengthened so that there can be more understanding by all of those involved as to the goals for a specific patient in the use of an art form?

2. Through this communication how can the attitudes of the dance or music or art therapist be coordinated with the over-all therapy and planning for a patient endowed with recognizable special talents?

The specific patients whom I will later mention are being used, not as being unusual nor as presenting individual problems, but rather as clear-cut examples of one problem shared by many. Both of these patients have the ability to dance better than the average person before constructive training in terms of their own self-expression, but not tremendous talent. Both have an intense interest in this form as a medium of communication. Both are considerably curtailed in making close and meaningful relationships, although they handle this difficulty in very different ways. Both have contributed in a useful way to the dance program during their hospitalization. Both are worthy of praise for their contributions to dance sessions and to the patients performances.

Neither young woman had had any appreciable amount of technical training before coming to the hospital, nor were they able to acquire any during their hospitalization, owing to a lack of interest in concentrating on technical work. Both were free and enjoyable to watch in their dance in the hospital setting. Because of their natural talent both have been encouraged to use the dance as a professional career on leaving the hospital by members of the staff unaware of the needs of such a career. One young woman is in her thirties and one is in her early forties. Even though she concentrated on developing knowledge and a technical skill to enable her to meet the demands of our present requirements as a performer in the dance, neither would be able to accomplish this in a period of time of less than from five to ten years. Yet both have been outstanding with their free forms of dance in the hospital setting, giving not only themselves but others pleasure through the use of dance.

If there is not an outstanding ability in performance the question of the use of this medium as a means of livelihood does not arise. The patient makes the use of the dance during his stay at Saint Elizabeths Hospital for which it was intended. This should also be the case of the people with an outstanding native ability. Many patients suggest that it would be fun to do dancing instead of office work after they leave the hospital. If they have attracted no special attention it is a simple matter to talk in terms of an amateur dance group or dance classes as an avocation and leave the dance as the fun it has been at the hospital. If, however, they have attracted special attention, it is not such a simple matter. This is where one feels the lack of needed communication and wishes that one were working toward common goals with other staff members. The patient is unable to hear me say that it would mean years of intensive training with no certainty of achieving a sure background of formal work to meet the competition. It is much more pleasant to be told that one could be a wonderful performer outside of the hospital as well as within it with no years of hard work. It is much more pleasant to hear that one is great through one's natural talent and that one could immediately be sought as a performer with much applause than to hear that after much study one might be a teacher of small classes.

It is simple for anyone unfamiliar with professional demands to fall into the trap of considering a dancer, a musician, an actor, or a painter outstanding in a setting where there is little material for comparison. Here self-expression in any of the arts is of prime importance. In the world outside of the hospital one starts instead of finishing with the asset of talent. There one must develop the skills of artisanship, achieved only through hours of intensive work. Within the hospital the artist is in an artificial environment where the best that one can do at the moment is accepted, where defeat is not permitted, where strivings are given support. Whether correctly or incorrectly, in the outside world the professional in the arts must be able to use a self-driven motor, must be accepting of criticism, must continue in spite of defeats and must accept and recognize his limitations. He is on his own all the way.

In suggesting or encouraging a patient to use the dance as a profession one is asking him to make use of stamina in a way that is frightening to the majority of people who have never been ill. The process of elimination is a cruel one. A person may be the best in a small school, but then he must be the best in the community, and then the best among hundreds in tryouts for one or two jobs. For a chorus line of ten or twelve there will be two to three hundred applicants, all good in many ways.

A patient can use the arts, whether in or out of the hospital, as a means of expression with considerable satisfaction, but I feel that great care should be used in suggesting professional use. Is it really supportive to encourage a patient to move into an area that requires so much in addition to his native talent? Should not great care be given to this with awareness of the personal requirements other than talent in an art form? Is this not an area of consultation between all of the disciplines, the social worker and the nurse as well as the doctor together with the leader in the art session? And in the end is it not better to leave the arts in the area of avocation where they have been satisfactory during the patient's stay at the hospital?

The patient whom I am presenting will not be present for interview, as I feel tht this would contribute nothing to the problems I am asking this conference to consider.

The patient who will be presented is Mrs. Dantur. She is no longer at Saint Elizabeths, having been discharged as recovered to the custody of the U. S. Marshal in 1959. Mrs. Dantur was admitted to Saint Elizabeths Hospital from prison where she had been serving a sentence since May 1950, in January 1953, with the diagnosis of Schizophrenic Reaction, Paranoid Type. She was extremely assaultive, restless, and bizarre in her actions and speech and began her hospitalization on one of the upper wards of the Women's Receiving Service. It was noted by the ward personnel that she spent some time each day in dancing to the radio music and it was suggested that I meet her and involve her in the dance sessions held in the dayroom of the ward. I met her during her first week in the hospital and her interest in the activities of the dance department continued until her discharge as recovered in June 1955.

Mrs. Dantur returned from prison in August 1955, after nine weeks out of the hospital and remained at Saint Elizabeths Hospital until she was again discharged as recovered to the custody of the Marshal in January 1959. At the time of her readmission she was "extremely perplexed and suspicious, misidentified others, had the feeling that she had been persecuted, and that doctors and guards were trying to kill her by putting poison in her food, and she was actively hallucinated in the auditory sphere."

Mrs. Dantur resumed her dancing almost immediately and continued to use this outlet throughout her stay until her discharge to prison in January of this year.

Mrs. Dantur's parents are living and have cared for her two children during the period of her hospitalization. They have visited her at intervals and occasionally have brought her children with them for short visits.

Mrs. Dantur was born in 1927 and was 26 years old at the time of her first admission to Saint Elizabeths Hospital.

She has one sister who is three years younger and married.

She has a brother who is eighteen months older.

The oldest sibling in the family died in childhood. The mother had a "nervous breakdown" after the birth of this child.

The family had a life that was very uncertain economically through the depression years. They moved frequently, owing to her father's loss of work and seeking of new employment. During one period they were forced to live in a cold water flat in crowded conditions. This shifting of residence caused a great deal of interruption to schooling. In spite of this, however, she was considered bright by her teachers.

During her childhood Mrs. Dantur was apparently the favorite of her father, while the sister and brother were favored by the mother.

Economic conditions improved at the time she entered high school. But it was at this time that she was observed to have difficulty with authority. Her absence from classes caused difficulty with the truant officer which led in 1943 to a truancy charge.

It was during this period that she was observed to show jealousy in competition with her siblings. She frequently ran away from home. She started at fourteen to take office work jobs during the summer months, lying about her age and returned to school only when forced to do so by the truant officer.

At sixteen she left home and supported herself by working as a model.

At seventeen, while still living away from home, she married a man in the service who was ten years older, but she did not introduce him to her family until a year later after the birth of her first child just prior to going overseas.

Her second child was born in Germany and she had two suicide attempts prior to the birth of this child. In speaking of this while she was at the hospital she stated that she had no other way out of a bad situation. Her religion forbade divorce.

She was talented in painting as well as dancing and used this medium of expression as well as the dancing throughout both hospitalizations. Her first use of painting was in the decoration of the walls of her room. Later, she used large sheets of wrapping paper on which she drew with crayons, the only available tools permissible on her ward. At this time her drawings were brilliantly colored, but her subject matter was immature, usually a stereotyped exotic figure with elaborate headdresses and costumes. This was typical of her own manner of dressing. When she was very disturbed she wore gaily colored, curious costumes of a very decorative nature. She continued this form of costume throughout her stay. Her dress was always exotic in a very bizarre fashion. Although she was neat her dress was as bizarre as it had been at the time she was using typical decorative devices. Her make-up was always exaggerated, suggesting a feline mask. She seemed to use the whole costume both as an attention-getting device and as a means of creating a barrier, aiding her in her isolation and increasing the distance other patients kept from her.

During her second hospitalization she had the advantage of working with an art therapist who guided her into the use of abstract forms for the expression of feeling. Much of the content in these paintings was similar to that in her dance improvisations.

She had had no previous training in dance, and while she had the ability to move well, her first interest as she worked with me was in usual rather pretty steps and movements. I worked with her and another patient who had studied dance prior to coming to the hospital in special classes. Mrs. Dantur did not absorb the technical work, but she became more free in her improvisations. She came to the dance room for sessions as soon as permission was given and she seemed to feel pleasure from her dancing.

At this time she continued to make only superficial relationships with other members of the group, using the dance for her own release of emotion but keeping to herself except when dancing.

She joined the group doing the production of "Cry of Humanity" and took one of the leading roles in both the dramatic action and the ballets.

The group accepted her ability as a dancer and willingly gave her the leading role which she performed magnificently. However, during rest periods and later in the dressing room at Hitchcock Hall, she remained by herself, with one of the young men in the group or me. Her mood swings were uncertain and she remained isolated from others in the group at all times except in actual performance. The other patients accepted her isolation.

Mrs. Dantur saw resident doctors for therapy during a large portion of her stay at the hospital during this period of hospitalization.

She was discharged after the final performance of the patient performance in June to prison and returned in August 1955.

After her readmission she resumed her dance activities almost immediately. She also joined the group which was doing a repeat performance of the "Cry of Humanity." At this time her relationship to the group remained very much as it had been on her previous hospitalization.

Both her activities in her painting with her art therapist and in the dance department increased. In 1956 her paintings were exhibited in the National Art for Handicapped Contest and in 1957 a group were exhibited at a psychiatric conference in Switzerland by her art therapist with the permission of the hospital.

During 1957 she worked with Miss Christrup as secretary in industrial therapy. She was able to sustain a continuing relationship with Miss Christrup.

She showed growth in her creative activities in the dance, not only having ideas for group dances but being able to organize the ideas in such a way that she was able to direct the group into a finished product which was presented in the spring show. However, she was at no time able to relate to the members of the group as people, but only as the means of carrying out her ideas. She constantly needed support in this area. She was also a co-director of a short but effective patient skit presented at the Dix Pavilion and at the William A. White Service. Her ideas for the entire holiday show in January of 1958 were accepted by the group of people who performed in this production. She wrote a one-act play and directed it, designed the costumes and the staging, and worked long and earnestly on some of the stage sets. She needed a great deal of support for such a large undertaking, but she completed the task.

During this year she willingly performed at numerous parties, designed and worked hard on ward decorations, and continued painting sessions with her art therapist. However, her relationships with people on her ward showed little improvement. She remained isolated from the majority, and few made any attempt to get even mildly close to her.

In January of 1958 she withdrew from the dance group with the statement that she wished to concentrate on some painting projects and would return at a later date. However, she did not withdraw from the dance area, nor break the relationship with me. She used the dance room for improvisation, borrowed records to play in her room, and invited me to look at her paintings. Some of her paintings were given to the dance room and are hanging there.

All of her art products, including the dance, are without technical structure and the content is of a very personal nature. They are spontaneous and represent emotional expressions—often of a bizarre nature.

During 1957 she was encouraged by other staff members to think in terms of using the dance professionally. This is where the problem I am presenting came into the picture. I was aware that she had no tools for meeting competition in the world outside of the hospital and even if she could concentrate on a technical foundation it would take ten years to achieve sufficient control to use her dance in performance. When she would talk with me I would point out that to work away from the hospital she would need a sound foundation in some school of movement. I pointed out that performing would be difficult, but that teaching might be possible after a considerable time had been spent in learning one of the present-day dance techniques. Directors would need a finished performer. Whether our desire for conformity is right or wrong, it exists. As director of a concert group I would need this, too. One does not have time to teach how to do a needed movement when one is directing a group composition. It would be too difficult to try for a performing career at nearly forty. Teaching could be done if she were willing to work very hard for a number of years. I also pointed out that joining some amateur group for an avocation would be fun. This she could never hear.

A structured class in basic techniques was started for her with five or six other patients for the purpose of finding out how she liked such a class situation. Her frustration tolerance was very low and dancing was not a pleasure to her in this situation even though the instruction was slow and fewer demands were made than in classes I hold outside of the hospital. Competition was painful to her and she quickly withdrew from the class.

During this period she was very tense because of an appeal of her case to the Supreme Court. In April she received news that her case was refused, became angry with me, and announced that she was throwing away her dance shoes. However, she placed them in the dance room before leaving the hospital without permission.

She was returned to the hospital later in the month. When she moved to Richardson Service she started a class with the patients in her building. She asked me for help which I gave her in encouragement to start, records, and a new pair of dance shoes. I have seen her only at intervals since April. Her greeting always is warm. An attendant brought her to the dance room to say "good-bye" and she has written me once from prison. In her letter she stated that she still wished to do dancing as a career.

I feel that much of her conflict about dancing and her inevitable defeat could have been avoided by strong and positive channelling into dance as an avocation rather than an expression of conflicting opinions by other staff members. Dance in free form is one of the few means for relating to others that she has been able to use. However, with her low self-esteem and low tolerance of frustration and defeat, is it possible for her to meet the competition in either painting or dancing as a career? The arts can be used by the majority of people as an avocation with great satisfaction. They can be used in this way for more successfully for real personal gratification.

Dance Therapy for Adults

The arts, whether painting, music, drama or dance, are well recognized as being of importance to people as a means for the communication of emotions or ideas that are difficult to translate into verbal forms. The dance, in particular, is perhaps more potent than any other of the art forms. Man lives his life in rhythm and expressive body action and these are the elements that are involved in dance whether the primitive religious forms or the social dances of today. As Dr. Joost A. M. Meerloo comments in "The Dance", "Man uses many forms of rhythm and dancing to reveal himself. While communicating with others he is involved in a continuous motoric interaction, moving toward and away from one another. In the unobtrusive dance of conversation people make minute gestures, they increase their stream of words and sound vibrations inadvertently, or use long silences while their rhythm of breathing changes."

When attention is focused on verbal interchange, the body action of the conversers passes unnoticed and is ignored as though it were non-existent. This is especially true in our culture where we rarely grant ourselves the privilege of giving vent to strong emotion. Nevertheless emotion breaks through the bonds of our strong controls. To quote John Martin in "The Dance", "Nature has so constituted us that movement is the medium in which we live our lives. The movements themselves actually have in them the essential nature of the emotional experience even though we have rationally directed them and they do not specifically 'mean' anything."

The essential aloneness that threatens people generally in our culture is augmented and increased by the distances we are able to maintain. Perhaps it would not seem so essential to us to maintain this distance if we dared to express our emotions directly, if we dared to share these with others rather than to hide them and converse in largely emotionless, neat comment. This would not matter so much if there were more frequent agreement between our verbal speech and our inadvertent body actions. Our real lives are lived in rhythm and movement, but we rarely share our true feeling. In a culture where distance between people is more usual than closeness, dance sessions become of paramount importance as a substitute for the natural spontaneous expression of emotion.

People who are patients in a hospital have exaggerations of the feelings of all people, but no difference in the feelings. Dance, then, is most valuable as a means of reducing the loneliness caused by these exaggerations of emotion and consequent increased separation from others.

Certainly, the adult overwhelmed with emotional problems reveals the extreme aspect of this isolation and consequent loneliness. He actually has one asset if the emotions he is revealing are not too overwhelming to others. Conversation is too effortful to participate in when it is concerned with other than his own feelings. These are usually too intense to speak about and consequently he remains alone expressing his separation from others in body action. He truly is living his life in movement, however much a defeated one.

Basic dance is perhaps one of the most effective means to cut through this isolation when the loneliness cannot be expressed in words, and the preoccupation with this emotion is too intense to converse about other matters. Even when a lack of initiative prevents a patient from joining a group moving together in rhythm the observation of such a group in rhymic action may make a bond which will cut through the distance maintained by the patient.

It is rare to conduct a session of dance on a ward of the hospital where the patients present are not either participating in the action or watching the session. All dance action expresses some emotion, joy, hate, peace, strength or defeat, and once an emotional experience has been shared a tenuous relationship has been established and the patient can be absorbed into the group of people who are sharing the rhythmic activity. Inherent in group rhythms is a strong, contagious fellowship. Again, to quote John Martin, "When and if a tribe performs a war dance, it is not exclusively for its mimetics influence over the enemy; it is also for the establishment of solidarity in the tribe." When one sees a group on a hospital ward performing rhythmic action together in the primitive circular formation one is intensely aware of the importance of this activity to the primitive tribe.

A positive quality of aliveness is present in the group of dancers which is in strong contrast to the patients who are sitting listlessly absorbed in no activity withdrawn from all others in loneliness. It is exciting to see one of these passively still people rise as though drawn by a magnet and move toward this living group. One must subscribe to the belief that rhythm and a shared emotional experience is important to a feeling of well being. Basic dance is the externalization of these inner feelings which cannot be expressed in rational speech but can only be shared in rhythmic, symbolic action.

If this feeling of solidarity in the group were all that happens in a dance session, it would be enough. However, there are many other facets of a positive quality as a group of people move together in rhythmic action. I have used the term people rather than patients advisedly. Dance action is useful in the hospital setting not because the patients are patients but because they are people. The same phenomenon of unity in a group of dancers together would be observable in any setting. It is only so striking in the hospital setting because a group cohesion is rarely observable. It is out of this shared experience of rhythm and expression of emotion that many other useful things can happen.

The question is often posed as to whether the physical activity is not the most important part of the dance session. If so, it would be equally effective for the group to participate together in calisthenics. Gymnastic exercise is very valuable and, without question, is an important aid in keeping physically fit, but it does not fulfill the same function that rhythmic action or dance achieves. Dance is not only important as physical exercise but it also involves the emotions through the symbolic movements. When the total person becomes a participant in an activity with other individuals it rarely seems important to stay removed from these other people. Changes of mood take place almost visibly and verbal conversation develops.

There should be no inference that the description of patients as being withdrawn and isolated means that they are all passive. I have been describing people with one outward aspect, but the patient is often overactive, restless and hostile. Talk is almost continuous and scattered. This does not mean any less isolation and loneliness but rather more. Conversation is almost an impossibility as it is too difficult to follow the rapidly changing mood swings. Verbal hostile attacks are more frequent than an attempt to meet the person trying to reach out in conversation. Only frustration can be the result, as this patient is using words to maintain distance, just as another may be using separation in space for this purpose.

Dance sessions are even more important for this patient than they are for the passive overtly withdrawn one. The physical activity takes care of his need for exercise and, since the majority of his emotional expressions are angry and aggressive, it is useful to him to be able to discover that the expression of these hostile feelings can be shared by others, rather than meet only retaliation, usually in the form of a withdrawal from him. There are few instances where his behavior is acceptable or where his actions do not bring retaliation. Whether it is the muscular relaxation through strenuous activity or the shared simple dance actions which can be interpreted as a symbolic expression of destruction there is a comfort in the relaxation that accompanies these rhythmic actions.

It is difficult to begin a relationship when almost the only way in which a patient can meet another person is with anger, sarcasm and hostility. In the majority of instances, the only possible reaction of the other person is one that leads to an active quarrel or a rapid withdrawal. This hostility can be met with symbolic battle in dance which will develop into a shared experience that often leads into the beginning of mutual understanding. Answering movement in similar forms dissipates his feeling of apartness, whereas a battle of words can only increase the feeling of closeness.

However, it is not only an expression of anger that is denied to people in our culture, but almost any observable emotion is looked at askance by the majority of people. Dispassionate conformity is considered the ideal behavior pattern for most situations. People are not at all perturbed to function with others who reveal no emotion whatsoever directly, but they are embarrassed to have contact with someone expressing strong emotion, either happy or sad. Dance action, then, in a hospital setting, is important for many reasons. Conversation can be ignored, but it is difficult to ignore a number of people joined together in a rhythmic activity. Not only are the people participating feeling a sense of belonging to a group, but there is a strong pull on the patients who are observing the action, particularly when it is performed in a circular formation. Again, to quote John Martin, "The group becomes one in conscious strength and purpose, and each individual experiences a heightened power as part of it." This feeling of a shared experience communicates itself to the observers, especially when it is mutually happy. Somewhere in any emotional experience the body enters. People sitting in isolation about the room are expressing this isolation with their posture and the intensity of tension in their musculatures. Whether it is shame, hostility or a general defeat that a patient is experiencing it is reflected in the musculatures of the various patients. Contrariwise the activity in the group is expressive of sureness, strength and harmony and this is translated into an emotion of a positive sort by the people who are either participating or watching. The change in the climate of the area in which the session is taking place can be visibly observed. Bodies that appeared weak and inadequate become stronger with vital action. Tension or indifference change to relaxation. Personal commitment to the sharing of an experience takes the place of a commitment to the maintaining of distance from people and a refusal to participate in anything going on with the demands for the assumption of responsibility, in other words, a personal involvement.

A technique for achieving this positive result is through simple rhythms in a circular formation. The rhythm must be constantly sustained throughout the session by the leader. Many patients move in ways which are rhythmic by usual standards. Since the patient uses little or no torso action, the movements are generally inadequate and awkward. However, if the leader adapts her movements to those of one of the patients who is involved in what she is doing, others can be led to follow, and a strong support is given to the patient who has initiated the particular movements.

The leader then develops the theme of the action using broader movement and involving sets of muscles, not used by the patient initiating the dance movement. During the course of the development of the rhythmic sequence, movements initiated by other patients expressing various moods are absorbed into the rapidly changing patterns. While it all seems a spontaneous flow of movement the leader is actually first joining one spontaneous expression in action and then another. From the time that the session begins until it ends, the leader is rarely forced to use her own ideas for the basis of the dance action, provided the ideas expressed in the group are accepted.

Another phase of the leadership of this sort of session is the constant flow of conversation. In the teaching of other people to lead such sessions this seems to be one of the most difficult parts of the technique for developing spontaneous involvement and personal commitment of the individual members. Dance sessions for the purpose of creating an activity which can help people to become interested require that the leader develop an ability in three directions. First, and most importantly, she must be able to sustain rhythmn throughout the session. Second, she must be able to speak in a way to create changes of mood. Third, she must be sufficiently secure to be constantly alert to the movements of the group with respect for them. The session should start slowly and gradually increase the tempo of their movements. During this section of the session, movements alternate between those expressive of mood and those which are directed toward improving coordination or achieving technical skills in various forms leading to better posture and walking ability. As a result there will be a general improvement in awareness of self and a consequent more ready acceptance of others with less fear. A good session can usually be evaluated as such by the laughter and lively conversation taking place between members of the group rather than with the leader, and the atmosphere of the ward will be one of relaxation.

Leadership in Dance Sessions Within the Institutional Setting

Dance is usually one of the most popular activities in mental hospitals. Programs run the gamut from social dances attended by large groups of patients to sessions with individual patients which are accepted as a part of the treatment program for re-socialization. All of these programs come under the name of dance therapy.

Recreation is needed if patients are not to remain isolated in little islands of aloneness. It is difficult for people who feel alone to join spontaneously in group activities without a great deal of urging from the workers on the staff. Ideas often cause intense distrust. Concentration is very nearly impossible and preoccupation with thoughts that are often disturbing prevent a free exchange with others. However, dance is an activity which can cut through these difficulties and be shared without too much overurging. This then becomes a shared experience involving both music and rhythmic body action which is often a happy one even for people who are essentially strangers.

Another advantage of dance is the fact that it is an activity in which volunteer workers can feel useful in the hospital situation. It there is to be a satisfactory interchange between the hospital and the community life outside of the hospital volunteer workers must feel that they are needed as an integral part of the hospital setting and that they can develop meaningful relationships while they are there. When people have intense emotional problems there are a number of reasons for them to have difficulty in being with others in a satisfying way, but dance can frequently help both patients and volunteers have satisfactory experiences while they are together.

Today, perhaps the greatest interest among those who are working with the people who need care in a hospital, is in a rapid social recovery for them and a return to life in the community. Consequently, the more the hospital community can remain a part of the larger community the more easily the patient can return to his former productive life. Volunteer workers are most important in keeping an active contact with the home community for the patient and contrariwise, an awareness of patients as part of the total community for people living outside of the hospital. The dance leader who is trained has an opportunity to develop an atmosphere in which these possibilities can be the core of the session which involves both volunteers and patients.

This implies the need for many qualities in the leader other than a liking for dance or highly developed technical skills. It implies an interest in basic body action and rhythms, an alertness to the possibility of communication through movement coupled with an interest in the people who are using this form of communication. In other words, to lead sessions in dance that are more meaningful than an enjoyable recreation requires interest, knowledge and skills that are more than technical proficiency in dance as a performer or an ability to teach.

First, as the leader, it is important to be willing to have not perfectionistic goals. This means shifting the accent from teaching dance as an art form to using dance skills in a way that will enable members of the group to relate to those involved in the activity through body action. This is very pat to say. It is less easy to do. It takes training in leadership and sincere interest in the functioning of others as people rather than an interest in technical dance forms. Teaching dance as an art form is very different from creating a climate in which patients dare to develop their own movements as sincere and real expressions of their emotions.

In the world outside of the hospital dance is sometimes a superficial display of technical skill which may be very beautiful, but often contains within the performance either a conscious divorcement from feeling or a stylized exaggeration of emotion. On the contrary, within the hospital, movement must always be sincere if it is to be therapeutic. All dance action should be related to daily activity.

Dance is an activity that is important as a means of expression to people whether they are well or ill only if it is meaningful both to the performers and to those sharing in the performance. Superficiality is not necessarily harmful to a patient, but nothing of value will happen and no group interaction with communication will occur during a session. Sincere expression through body action is even more important in the re-education of people who are again beginning to live than it is in the education of children.

When a person is essentially distrustful of others, the development of a relationship is a slow process. A patient will test another person again and again before believing that the other person is worth trusting. On a verbal level this is a very slow process, especially in group sessions, whereas sharing rhythmic action often speeds up this process. It is impossible to share this experience without a certain amount of rapport developing. While this understanding may need to be reestablished on the next meeting, it is helpful to have had it established the first time and can be the first step toward other interaction. It often creates a climate which will enable a patient to be free enough and sufficiently confident in the people around him to express real feeling both on a positive and a negative side with a sense of belief that he will be understood. Consequently, much attention has been given in the last few years to the use of body action as a group activity with hospitalized mental patients.

The second important attitude of a leader of dance sessions in a hospital setting is that of seeing his role as that of someone functioning with the group as a person rather than as a performer. Understanding or awareness of a patient as a person is the thing that he needs perhaps more than anything else. Nobody can like prickly behavior nor is it useful to a patient to have a pretense of acceptance by others. But in the relaxed atmosphere of sessions of rhythmic movement the behavior that has a tendency to alienate others can often be discarded by the patient, at least temporarily.

If the leader accents his performing ability and arouses admiration for his technical dance ability, he will defeat his main purpose of developing in the patient group confidence in themselves. Since communication through body action is the focal point of the dance sessions, there should be no need felt by the leader to perform, but rather to foster creative movement in the patients as individuals and as a group. Since they have intense lack of confidence in themselves and in each other there must be a feeling of acceptance of their abilities before a climate can be developed in which they can feel comfortable. This is the function of the leader.

Another attitude of the dance leader must be one of simple directness. Patients who are insecure are very alert to oversweetness. There is nobody who likes flattery. Immediate distrust develops between people because of flattery. Unfortunately, patients often believe that a sincere feeling of appreciation of their achievements is only flattery. The leader must be able to sense when to compliment at rare intervals and when merely to accept.

When young people think of entering the field of dance with mental patients they must be willing to think in terms of the development of the simple abilities of the patients. So long as a person wishes to perform dance for an audience he should realize that he is not ready to use dance as a tool for resocialization with mental patients.

There is no greater satisfaction than that of seeing confidence and initiative develop in someone who has been lacking in this. But it is a satisfaction far removed from the satisfaction in a good piece of work in dance composition or dance performance.

Rhythmic Action for Communication

Communication that is meaningful, too frequently is either impossible or inadequate. Distance between people is the more expected and often the more acceptable situation. The acculturation process in this culture starts at a very early age. Owing to the word centered culture in which we live, it is often expected that the only useful communication will be on a verbal level. The emotional level of communication, which is a needed exchange between people, to cut through isolation, is "tabu". This situation is to be found even among members of a family or between intimate friends. The fact that there are two levels of exchange (verbal and emotional) is ignored. It is as though people are unaware that they are always communicating on the non-verbal level. Even though they remain silent verbally, they never stop communicating on the non-verbal level.

Frequently, emotions are so close and meaningful to a person, that there must be a tool for communication that does not require the use of words. It is often important that the emotion expressed remain on the less threatening non-verbal level. It is also true that people with intense emotional problems find the need for communication on the non-verbal level more necessary than people with less pressing problems.

Art forms often fill this need. Although the use of an art form is different for mental patients than it is for an artist, perhaps patients have an even greater need for an art expression than the community at large. Especially, in their use of symbolic movement rather than words as a customary way of functioning, is this so. However, the arts are needed as a means of non-verbal communication whether used by people in the community or in the hospital setting.

Patients always use art forms for direct expression on the non-verbal level. Sometimes this is a release of emotional tensions without the intention of a purposeful communication with another person. But if there is empathy with this other person, the patient will accept a sharing of this non-verbal expression and direct communication results.

The patient never attempts to refine his concepts, but leaves his use of the art form as a direct expression of his intense emotions. Consequently, it lies outside of art as such and remains a valuable means for expression of feeling and, only occasionally, when shared, a direct communication.

One asset of people with emotional problems is the fact that they use physical action to express feeling more readily than the majority of people in our culture who are so constricted in this direct expression. The tragedy is that the emotions which they are expressing are often not acceptable to the community at large whether in or out of the hospital.

Even when these feelings are logical, patients cannot believe that they will be understood. Consequently, they continue to feel isolated unless their non-verbal expression is answered with understanding. Therefore, to be involved in a group action where the expression of any feeling is not only acceptable but a shared experience is an important facet of dance therapy. Sessions of dance therapy even use action that is basically hostile. Patients fear the destructive force of their naturally aggressive as well as hostile feeling. Out of these moments expressing aggression or anger, members of the group can then express warmth without a concomitant overwhelming fear. How much better it would be if members of the community could experience this sharing of emotion. However, this cannot happen while people hold themselves apart from expression of feeling in a restricted way and communicate only verbally. However, this can be understood easily when one is aware that even young children are taught to be self contained and restrained.

It is unfortunate that the way in which people express feeling at any given moment is largely unknown to them. When it is impossible to ignore strong feeling, words often are used to disguise these feelings. However, words are worse than useless. The real feeling already has been expressed in action. Words can be controlled, facial expression can also be disguised in some ways, but the small unconscious muscle tensions around the eyes and the mouth reveal what is going on. The tone of voice is also as difficult to control as other small muscle tensions.

Actually, however, I am not talking about facial expressions, or any other piece of body action. I am speaking of a person as a whole. Unconscious muscle contractions throughout the body are constantly expressing feeling. Dance therapy is making use of the communication that is constantly occurring between all people.

Some people are very expressive of feeling. Warm greetings of friendship, body action expressive of impatience and anger are expected from them. However, the majority of people are self-constrained and inhibited in these physical expressions of emotion. Usually, others present are embarrassed by the people who express their feelings freely and openly.

Since words are used as disguise or denial, almost more frequently than to communicate directly, the forming of meaningful relationships requires that both levels—the verbal and the non-verbal—must be involved and compatible. When this happens, true interaction occurs. However, one serious hindrance to this is the fact that everyone has a tendency to feel as though he were behind a one way mirror. For interaction, however, all people need to express emotion as well as to use verbal speech. People seem to feel a hesitancy in revealing themselves. They apparently feel defenseless, as though it would be destructive to them to reveal who they are at all times.

If this would be useful in the community, it is even more necessary in the hospital or clinic setting. Here relationships are frequently established on a non-verbal level by empathizing with the communication of the patient's expression of feeling in movement.

Dance therapy is making use of the most basic movements expressive of emotion. While in dance therapy rhythm is added, the actions are those used by everyone. Although these are often out of their awareness, these are often brought into awareness in shared symbolic rhythmic action. It is used, therefore, as a therapeutic tool for communication and body awareness in institutions, clinics and special schools. Even where physical difficulties are the most obvious problem, the basic techniques of movement for communication are still the principal base of dance therapy. Physical difficulties often lead to emotional problems and therefore awareness of expression of feeling is needed. In a way, "dance" is a misnomer for dance therapy unless one accepts the term "dance" on the most basic level. It is sometimes confusing to the majority of people, as they frequently have preconceived and often superficial concepts of dance. A better, although more clumsy, expression would be emotional communication in body action.

While all forms of art are useful for expressing feeling, dancing and singing have the added value of involving the use of the individual's own body in these forms of non-verbal communication. They are the best means for directly relating.

Dance therapy is used in all areas of the hospital, since it is as important to those who function in a flat stereotyped way as it is for those who do not function well but who are spontaneous as well as expressive.

Dance therapy is not the only group interaction where non-verbal communication occurs. Even in verbal therapy, it is essential that the leader be aware of all that is taking place on other levels than the verbal, if full use of the emotional expression is considered.

Even where the therapist is uninvolved verbally, he cannot remain uninvolved with body action. He will respond without awareness, but it would be useful if he could acknowledge his emotions to himself even though he did not impose these feelings in a directive way on the group. Only in this way can the two levels of communication (verbal and emotional) continue as parallel means of recognition of others as people.

Since non-verbal expression is always present, it is useful for people in the community as well as in the hospital to recognize what is going on.

When Expressive Therapy In The Dance Is Contra-Indicated

It is perhaps an heretical idea to suggest that there are times when direct expression of an emotion by a patient in any of the aesthetic forms is contraindicated. Since non-verbal communication in an art form is often the only means open to a withdrawn patient, it would seem that any personal expression in cutting through his isolation would be of value. One usually speaks of the instances where this is the case when talking or writing about the use of the arts with mental patients, and in doing so, too often sounds as though the complete answer for a patient comes through the expression of emotion in an art form.

Expression through the arts for a mental patient is usually a very direct one, and therefore occasionally it would seem to be contra-indicated, at least in dance action or body movement. Painting and music have an end product that is outside of a person except for the act producing it.

Dance, on the contrary, involves the individual in the end product and contains the elements for a direct communication of the emotions. This makes it more potent in its affect than verbal communication. One of the difficulties encountered in transposing an emotional experience into verbal terms is that much of the intensity and awareness in an individual of the implications in an experience are lost in speaking or writing of it.

The artist performer or choreographer must develop an initial idea into objective terms. This is a parallel process to that of speaking of an emotional experience. While basically his composition contains all of the elements of direct communiction in movement, it does not stop at this. Whether he is presenting a formal abstraction in designed action or a dance intended to arouse an emotional response in his audience, he must not remain subjectively and personally involved in his compositon to the exclusion of the world around him. In other words, he does not remain subjectively involved in communicating his fantasy. One can say that the artist is self conscious or self aware or that he uses an international form in his performance or composition. In other words, he has removed himself as a person absorbed in the emotions of certain movements and has added an intellectual component, a highly critical evaluation.

I can remember how strongly Ruth St. Denis stressed in her teaching that a person must look at his favorite composition, the thing most tenderly loved at the moment, and throw it away because somehow it has failed. Only then can he begin to understand the meaning of work as an artist. One cannot deny that this viewing and critical appraisal of a piece of work is subjective but both the intellect and the emotions of the person are involved. Consequently, this attitude is based on a knowledge of body action, the rules of composition, and the awareness of the impact of the direction of a body or bodies through space on an audience. This enables the individual to become objective.

It is out of this combination of the emotional and intellectual involvement that drama is created for an audience by such great performers and choreographers as Martha Graham, Harald Kreutzberg or Jose Limon in the field of modern dance, and John Kriza, Jerome Robbins or Agnes deMille in the field of contemporary ballet. The artist always continues to refine and to make more concise and more formalized his composition long after the first showing for an audience. This change from the subjective involvement in a dance to an objective presentation is a difficult if not an impossible task for a psychotic patient and one not comprehended by him. There is no doubt that a great deal is said by patients in their compositions, but it is nevertheless a direct communication far removed from the objective approach of the artist. Even though their compositions are not improvisations in the theater, nevertheless, they remain on a subjective level.

The compositions of the schizophrenic patient are a direct statement of his particular emotion of the movement. The very fact that he is freed by his illness to express his feelings in movement makes his expression of them far more exciting in some ways than the formal, technically aware composition of the self conscious or self aware artist performer. He rarely concerns himself with a development or modification of his original idea. He concerns himself not at all with whether his initial form could be made stronger by lengthening or shortening the dance, by changing the movements to bring sharper emphasis to certain sections of his composition or to the lines of emphasis that could be useful from a staging point of view. In addition, it would not occur to him to work on more technical proficiency for the purpose of presenting his idea with more clarity. Balance is totally lacking in his composition and the conclusion drawn out endlessly or chopped off with no apparent thought.

The complete idea must remain as first improvised or composed, no matter how many suggestions in the form of direction or coaching are given.

On the other hand he is very true, as a child is true, in his concepts of the emotions he wishes to express. He is more direct than the person who is less than the great artist. Consequently, he would never be guilty of presenting a dance that was a technical display without feeling. He would always dance his personal feelings of the moment rather than divorcing himself from them for the sake of dance in pure form.

This vast chasm between the expression of the psychotic patient and the artist becomes even more clear when one sees the approach within the same group which is composed of patients in contact with reality and those out of contact in varying degrees. Those patients who are in contact with reality follow the pattern of artists in the outside world. They also move from the subjective to the objective point of view in their performance as well as in their composing.

One such composition concerned the building of a Russian satellite. The form, staging, climax and conclusion were well thought out. The ballet not only had emotional impact, even giving a sense of fanatical worship, but it was based on a clear cut form which was structurally sound. This dance could be critically viewed and improved both as to form and an augmenting of the original intention.

In sharp contrast to this well structured composition was the ballet of the struggles of the emotions of Dorthea Lynde Dix which aroused much comment in audiences who saw it.

Even the music in this ballet was chosen by the patients to arouse the emotions in themselves which they wished to express. It is true that they were clear enough in their intentions to state in the dance what these emotions were. Nevertheless, the value lay in the impact on the audience of these emotions communicated in the raw, rather than from the building of a composition out of movements that would arouse feeling in people viewing it. This sort of subjective performance can be even more powerful at times than that of the performer who is objective and who begins with the emotions but who builds a powerful formalized pattern for the purpose of an intentional communication.

The artist emphasizes the emotional feeling, the self awareness and with thought pulls together all of these elements into what he believes and hopes will make a good piece of work. This combined with a self conscious awareness of how to achieve his purpose, as he views it, causes him to develop that quality known as style so that we recognized in a given piece of work the hand of a Doris Humphrey or that of an Agnes deMille. Contrariwise, the schizophrenic often has flair but never style. He has not concerned himself with the techniques which induce him to develop.

It is because of this lack of objectivity, this direct communication without intellectual artifice that dance is so valuable as a means of communication to the mental patient. Since he always dances out his feelings he frequently expresses emotions which are a part of his involvement in the distortions which he sees as real. In the majority of instances this is extremely useful to him. A patient in a mental hospital can rarely speak verbally about intense emotions. In spite of the schizophrenic's use of symbolism in words and his great facility in using language that relates divergent ideas which often makes his speech seem to have the quality of poetry, he does not communicate to others too well in this form. He also uses speech as a defensive tool as frequently as he uses it to communicate with others.

He does, however, communicate directly with movement, especially to a person moving with him at the moment, and often to an audience observing him. While this is usually an asset, there are times when the intensity of the emotion expressed or the rapidity with which he speaks of feelings close to him causes him to be frightened by the things he has clearly expressed. The leader in a dance session or the observer of an individual dance improvisation should be ready to control the situation and lead the patient into closely structured forms which contain little or no connotation with emotional expression.

Mr. N is a good musician who is very sensitive to rhythm and plays well enough to give pleasure to an audience. He is gentle and courteous towards others. He does not see qualities as assets, however, since he seems to envy a brother of whom he frequently speaks. Mr. N's brother was successful in playing football at school and at the present time is successful in the competitive field of business. Mr. N thinks of his brother as having the proper masculine abilities, while his own assets seem valueless to him since he thinks of them as being nonmasculine and consequently liabilities.

Dance improvisation to music which he has chosen, occasionally is sought by Mr. N when he has experienced some defeat or when he is feeling a great deal of tension. In his improvised dance action, he expresses an expansiveness that he rarely shows in his functioning in other areas. He is very often constricted in his movements and usually finds it difficult to relate to others even superficially and in the most formal way.

On the other hand, when he is dancing an improvisation he becomes relaxed,his coordination is smooth and his face lights up. However, he expresses the same side of his personality that is to the forefront when he is playing improvisations on the piano. This is the part of him that is not like his brother and which he distrusts. Mr. N will want to become involved in body action at other times but it would be very anxiety provoking to lead him into improvisation unless he himself seeks it out. He knows that I will give him instruction in strenuous gymnastic exercises that will help him to feel more adept in his body action and more masculine unless he indicates a wish for something else.

There is a great distinction between the creative dance and the technical area that leads to motor skill or body awareness for the patient. Free creative expression is based on direct communication and does not have the same goals as those of the artist. Consequently, the controls of translating the free expression into objective terms are lacking.

Learning body control is related to many things such as body awareness, pride in achievement and further adeptness in coordination which can be used in other areas. It is also related to the dance, but it is not creative in the sense of being a subjective expression. The session can be kept within these limits or shifts can be made between creative forms and structured technical instruction. There are occasions when the emotions expressed are so close to the patient, or they are so involved with his frightening ideas, that it is inadvisable to encourage recreative improvisation for periods of time.

Miss A had many body feelings of weakness and muscle inadequacy. She combined wishes to be a part of the group with "acting out" which was always in rebellion against conformity and authority. She was extremely verbal and was involved in expressing ideas of life and living. She had some awareness and curiosity in a way that is similar to any young woman of twenty, but her ideas also involved concepts that were peculiarly her own. In body action she had a feeling of satisfaction only when she was working to bring certain groups of muscles into play. If the leader had demanded that she express ideas in dance form, whether her own or those of the leader, she would not have been able to move. By apparently working only with the body and its muscle structure she could be led away from her verbal dissertations and into a freedom of action that was mildly creative even though within a rigid and apparently emotionless structure. Since she was unable to express feelings from herself at this time, she would have returned to her diffuse verbal pyrotechnics, if an attempt had been made to direct this into creative expression.

Another patient, Miss Y, was strongy involved in morbid ideas of death and destruction. She had factually seen death as a solution for severe problems at one time and had killed her husband. Her dances in a creative form led inevitably to this point during one psychotic episode. In combining her creative ideas into a structured form for teaching other people a group dance based on her ideas she was able to relate to others for the first time during her hospitalization. The creative dance was the basis for this structuring, but by centering her thinking on the patterns of her ideas for the group to carry out, her intrest was aroused in structured forms which were outside of her subjective morbid emotion. Here the creative art was useful, but only with the addition of having to teach and therefore forced her to make her ideas objective rather than a totally direct communication of her morbidity in an exaggerated form.

Some patients are able to keep a superficial control which makes them seem more "put together" than they are. This surface control is very thin and if it cracked obviously would leave the patient in panic with nothing to hide behind. For people like this, all manner of forms of structured physical action is useful in giving them a well developed physical control. This can help them begin to feel themselves as "put together" people in a real sense.

It is essential that the leader of movement sessions be aware of when the encouragement of creative forms is useful and when the closely structured formal pattern with no individual expression is most helpful to patients. At all times non-verbal communication exists between the leader and the patients whether working in the area of structured sessions for body control or in the area of free emotional expression.

When alertness to the varied needs of the patients is developed by the dance leader, he can easily determine when sessions of dance in a creative form are indicated or when sessions of structured body exercises are most useful.

1. Dance as a means of communication in a free creative form is always useful for the passive regressed patient.
2. Dance as a creative art form is highly useful to the patient who is seeking an outlet for emotions about which he finds difficulty in speaking.
3. Dance as a creative art form is contra-indicated for the tense stereotyped patient. It is essential to help him gain body control and muscle relaxation through non-emotional structured forms of exercise.
4. Dance in a creative form should be alternated with highly structured sessions for the patient who becomes over excited or panicky from his emotional expression.

I have made a distinction between creative forms of dance and structured forms of body control. I believe that even teachers of dance and dancers themselves often fail to make this distinction. It is essential to make this differentiation in the hospital setting.

Talk for Louisiana State Community Ballet Group Conference

The State of Louisiana is to be congratulated on the encouragement of the community ballet groups. The organization has not only given support within the state, but has been a strong enough organization to cause the membership to grow thoughout much of the Eastern seaboard and to other communities as far away as Oklahoma. The growth of this movement negates the attitude that the arts should be looked upon as something to be used and participated in by small groups endowed with special gifts of talents in the community in general. It is through this broad participation that those with special aptitudes will be able to have support and encouragement from a very early age, while at the same time many others will have enjoyment.

I am not sure whether the concept of education and appreciation of the art form of ballet were the only reasons for the support of the community groups, or the major one, but, nonetheless, this Association has been, is, and will be responsible for many other aspects in the development and growth of the young people at a most needed time in history.

Dance is one of the best media for communication between people. It is doubly important in this period when people need to have understanding for one another, but, more frequently than not, feel very isolated. One reason for the loneliness of individuals in our culture is the lack of the means to communicate on an emotional level in a culturally accepted form. All art forms, whether painting, drama, literature, or music, furnish outlets for expression of and communication of emotion. Music and dance, however, as the social arts, are the most potent forms for the sharing of feeling.

At one time in the history of man all in the village would be involved in producing art forms, without concern for relative artistic merits and the efficiency of various individuals producing these forms, but only concern with what was being said. Villages were rich in these art products. It was taken for granted that as man could speak thoughts, so could he give expression in other ways on the many levels of himself as a person.

As we became more and more intellectualized, the use of the arts became less a natural expected expression from people but was left to specially gifted artists. A painting must be worthy to be hung in a gallery or it is a waste of time to make a painting. Music must be worthy to be performed in concert by other musicians before anyone will attempt a composition. Dance, too, the most important need of man, for the most part has become a spectator diversion.

You have not gone back to the primitive, you have combined our present need for knowledge and demand for technical perfections in a most demanding and highly developed form of dance, with encouragement for participation rather than passive observation. You are meeting the needs of the growing and developing young person and, at the same time, setting standards for appreciation for especially skilled performers.

Since the beginning of history it is known that man has used dance for individual and group expression of feeling. There are many emotions that cannot be put into words. Whether we spontaneously give expression to passing emotions in movement or we use movement consciously in a dance form, these are both ways in which we convey these feelings. Ballet is a complex form of skills for the clear expression of the feelings of man, as well as the development of special skills.

In developing the technical skill for this clear expression, the person becoming able to be a master of the art is developing his body coordination to a remarkable degree. This, too, is an asset to the developing young person. As he becomes adept and fine coordinations are mastered, he knows himself better. In being aware of a straight spine and the functioning of his arms and legs and head, the student becomes more aware of himself as a person. When one is more aware of himself he can relate better to others.

In other words, you are not only furthering the art of the dance and developing more knowledgeable and appreciative young people, but you are causing these young people to be more aware of themselves and others, one might say developing better citizens.

Dance is closely allied to the nonverbal forms of communication which everyone unconsciously uses together with the verbal, but on which the acutely ill mental patient who is often inarticulate is almost totally dependent.

Basic dance, then, either in group or as an individual expression, is especially well adapted for use, as an adjunctive therapy of acutely ill psychotic patients, where communication is more restricted than among people in general.

The contemporary dance has consciously concerned itself with an attempt to understand the response of the body to inner emotions. It has also developed varying techniques to channel these movements into direct expression. The term "basic dance" has been coined to differentiate it from the artificial and elaborate forms of dance which depend upon physical "tours de force" as a means of entertainment, rather than communication.

The acutely ill, regressed schizophrenic patient, is largely cut off from the means of communication which are open to others in his environment. He makes use of his body action to convey his emotions. Stripped of the usual repressions of our word-centered culture, he is able to use his body with extraordinary directness and clarity in dance forms which are often closely parallel to those of the modern dancer. Both groups make use of symbolization in body action. While the modern dancer uses them for communicating an idea to a particular audience, and the schizophrenic patient uses them for giving expression to autistic emotion, they both arrive at remarkably similar forms.

One young man used the entire floor space available to him in his day room to dance a formal processional. His body control was superb and there was no superfluous movement. His entire body was involved in stylized motions expressive of grandiose power. He alternated this with the most abject grief as he sank to the floor as if he wanted to bury himself in it. As he had not used verbal communication for many weeks, I was asked to dance with him, to form a relationship, if possible. At the time of our first meeting, I was convinced that he must have been a pupil of Harald Kreutzberg. Many of the gestures he used were identical with those of the German dancer. He accepted my dancing with him and after six or seven sessions, he spoke to me. He was able to tell me that he had never studied dancing in any form. At this time he spoke mostly of the delusion that he was God, which he alternated with expressions of deep hopelessness, as he had in his dance.

Because I had moved with him in his expression of feeling, he was able to feel that I understood him. After a period of time he was able to speak, and, because we had shared his ideas through the dance, he was able to give verbal expression to the same ideas. In other words, we knew each other.

As he used more and more verbal expression, his bizarre ideas were modified. We also shifted in our dancing and were eventually doing ordinary ballroom dancing. By then, too, we were having interesting conversations about art and literature.

This, of course, is only one use of dance with a patient.

One characteristic of modern dance is its concern with the dancer in space. The schizophrenic patient by his very self-containment makes one aware of the space that he is not occupying. The manic-depressive patient makes extraordinary use of he space in which he moves. He withdraws from the environment or moves out into it with an acute awareness that seems to concern itself with space above and below him, as well as the plane on which he is moving. Any concert dancer might well envy him his mastery of this element in action. He seems aware of no limitation as he dances. He expresses his rapidly changing emotions with directness and clarity and in understandable terms.

The person who is experiencing a manic phase of the manic-depressive psychosis uses body action effectively and directly, either to augment his verbal communication or to reveal his underlying emotional reponse of the moment. This emotion often appears to be one of hostility caused by a feeling of restraint from authority figures or restrictions of his environment. The quick, impatient movements, similar though exaggeraed, to those anyone might use, and the need to move into space, even though someone or something is in the way, often causes needless retaliation. It has been my experience that patients use this aggressive behavior pattern as an expression of their feeling of the moment rather than toward an individual.

The ability to use movement as an expression of emotion in a direct way, together with his command of space about him, makes the manic patient an exciting and stimulating dancer. His movements are exaggerated, strong, beautifully coordinated dance motions, but they always appear to be expressions of anger, destruction, and despair. He seems to have no mental image of himself as successful, but only as reaching, attacking, and then despairing. When the dancer is left alone to complete his improvisation, he inevitably finishes it on the floor in a posture of self-degradation. Even though he physically tires himself, and in spite of the discharge of a great deal of emotional and physical energy, he seems to feel no relaxation. He continues to shout and is restless, with no lessening of difficulties with people in his environment.

During the process of re-socialization, this means of communication is gradually repressed until the patient moves with rigidity and over-restraint as he leaves the hosptial. Miss H expressed this feeling by saying, "I have learned to suppress my real emotion, but in doing so, I have reinforced my basic guilt feelings."

Dance is one form of action which can be used when a patient is very quick, excited, and unpredictable. Someone dancing with such a patient can also move quickly and express changing emotions. But one thing I have always been consistent about—I have always danced the role of a defeated person. If I did not, the patient will suddently give up his real feelings and will become an obedient, childlike person. But after dancing defeat and allowing the patient to conquer, he can then usually accept the authority of the leader, as well as dance with a group in a relaxed way and with what seems like acceptance and enjoyment.

One characteristic of the movement of the schizophrenic patient makes it seem more bizarre to the onlooker than perhaps it actually is. He seems to use only his hands, feet, and head to express his feelings. This creates movments which seem distorted to those of us who use our whole body. His withdrawal from the space about him also seems unnatural to us. Once one has accepted those two characteristics of his movements, however, he no longer seems strange and non-understandable. As one moves with him in his fashion rather than one's own, it is startling to discover how very direct he is being and how little he is making any attempt to hide his fear, guilt or hostility. An added factor brought into the picture in moving with a patient who is absorbed in fantasy, is the predominant one of isolation. To speak of the isolation of an actually ill schizophrenic patient becomes almost a cliche. It makes understandable his lack of any overt attempt to relate to those about him. He is unable to communicate his feelings in intelligible verbal terms and those about him are often too repelled by his direct communication in movement to attempt to understand.

He is also revealing through his movements his feelings of helplessness and dependence. It is not strange, then, that he seems to get no relief from anxiety through his posturings when he receives no satisfactory answer from those about him, on a level which he can accept. He seems to be lost in a four-way dearth of communication. The patient is expressing himself verbally in ways which do not communicate for the most part, but saying things directly in ways which are ignored, while those about him are speaking verbally in ways which do not reach him and expressing feelings of which they are unaware. Some of the bewilderment concerning people who are very sick must come from these four-ways means of communication which never meet.

I think it is through the attempt to move with patients in forms similar to theirs that has caused many of them to say, "You have known me from the beginning," and others to state, "Nobody wants to be alone." These remarks say clearly, "You answered me in movement when that was my speech."

Although the bizarre actions of mental patients are well recognized as protective mechanisms, they seem frequently to be attempts to communicate which are ignored.

I believe dancing in symbolic forms for the schizophrenic patient has an important aspect, when it is a shared experience. Since these feelings of guilt, overdependency and loneliness are too overwhelming to put into verbal terms, but can be directly expressed in movement, it follows logically that they must be answered satisfactorily to the patient to prevent further withdrawal into his isolation.

It is during the dancing in the circle that the withdrawn, usually motionless patient, is drawn into the activity and will even be able to join in the verbal conversation which develops at this time.

Miss C. danced her own improvisations for several sessions before she was able to join the group. On the day she joined the group she said, "I have been saying one thing. Now I am ready to talk with others about many things."

Occasionally, withdrawn patients may use the rhythmic action of the circular dance group as support while they continue to dance by themselves. Mrs. D. is withdrawn from the other patients on her ward for the greater part of the time. She remains curled up in a corner of the room absorbed in her own feelings. Occasionally she is obviously responding to hallucinations. She is unable to tolerate close contact with the members of a dance session as yet.

However, as the dance begins to absorb the majority of patients on her ward, and group patterns begin to develop, Mrs. D follows these rhythmic patterns with her eyes, her face becomes relaxed, and she responds with body movement to what is happening in the room.

Suddenly, after a large circle has been formed, she begins a rhythmic stamping movement of her feet which carries her around the room just outside of the circle of other dancers. As she stamps, she moves her shoulders forward with alternate sharp jerks, reaching with her arms as she chants, in time to the music, about her loneliness and isolation from others.

Dance therapy, in making use of the basic form of communication, offers the individual a means of relating himself to the environment or to other people when he is cut off in the majority of areas by the patterns of his illness.

His meaningful, though bizarre movements become understandable and acceptable to others as people relate themselves to him on the basis of the emotions expressed through dance action. As his feelings of isolation and his fear of a lack of understanding are reduced, he is able to put aside autistic expression to an increasing degree, and this, in turn, seems to enable him to enter a group and function within it in a manner that is satisfying both to the patient himself and to others in the group.

Dance therapy is first a method for initial contact and then support. It is a warming-up medium in which a patient becomes more aware of himself as an entity functioning with other entities in comparative safety.

Audio-Taped Discussion—Body Image

Specific relationship between body image, the world, and the personality:

When things work well you come out with a body image that is in tune with, related to, the reality of the world and the healthy aspects of the personality. And the body image is a true one. It coincides more with what the body actually looks like, what the mental image of the body is, and what the world looks at you as.

eg. When pathology gets into the picture this is where things become distorted. The person who is always pulled back from other people. Why? Because they don't believe other people have a true picture of them. They don't feel the people have a meaningful awareness of them.

They feel people see them in a way that is not acceptable. The person does not accept himself and he believes he is therefore unacceptable to others.

So the receding body image says—if I pull myself in or back, my body image recedes so I can disappear into space and it won't be so unpleasant, or I won't expose myself in an unpleasant fashion to others and to be judged.

eg. With autistic children even this does not take place because there is not a loss of body image, they have just never had a body image. They have had no relating experiences by which to learn or develop their body image. They have not been able to come into contact with reality to find out what is there, where they fit into the picture, or even to locate themselves in space.

What motor coordination autistic children have is not spatially oriented to themselves. It's more they are not aware of themselves doing it. It just happens. Its mostly just a physiological, neurological development that carries on within their own pace.

Therapeutic goals through rhythmic and body movement would work toward primarily an acceptance or an awareness of the person working with them. It would be much later you would work with them toward acceptance of themselves, because their selves is non-existant. Here you work toward having the autistic person identify with the dance therapist, and the therapist accepts this identification. This is not usually true in other therapeutic circumstances. The therapist would not work toward having the patient identify with the therapist This would not be a healthy result. Identification is part of the developmental pattern of acquiring a normal body image. What you do with autistic children is then go back through the developmental pattern in a rhythmic movement session. With the autistic you go back completely to the infantile developmental stages, working through them as the child is ready and capable of so doing.

And, at first, there is not a differentiation (on the part of the patient) between the body of the person with whom you are identifying and your own. Therfore, if there is an acceptance of you with the autistic child, there will be no differentation between that person and yourself. You don't necessarily work for this, it more just being aware this is what will happen. This is not a case of the therapist trying to lose her identity into that of the child. It is the reverse. If acceptance takes place it is because the autistic person has made the identification.

Once this identification has happened there is still no body image within the child, but you are now able to work slowly toward differentiation of the body images. You work with the autistic person's natural movements, enlarging them, broadening them—yet taking the leadership in movement from the patient. You take the followership. If you have the patient always in the position of following they will never differentiate. At first, though, they do have the followership. You recognize and follow their spontaneous leadership movements that they display as they are initially following the therapist's movements. This is a gradual and fluctuating exchange of leadership. You find out the person's leadership movements by taking their limited forms of movement "out" for a moment to see if they are ready for it. You test in brief flashes broadening their movements to determine how the patient does it, then you switch and follow how they are doing it.

e.g. If the autistic has a quality of movement that can be related to a specific, reality oriented movement (like guitar playing) you take that movement and begin using it for a specifically related purpose. Having the whole group (if you are working with a group) try the reality-oriented movement. It then becomes a functional movement, not just random finger movements in an infantile way.

You do this with movements also from people displaying different emotional disorders than autism. You take what they are doing and move it into a reality-oriented, functional expression. This is a basic aspect of movement therapy—one of its major goals. You try to transcribe aimless movements over into something that has meaning rather than aimless doing.

If the person does not accept the group's going into his movement he may change his own movement. You do not then switch to the new movement. This puts the person too much in the "spotlight". You carry on into something else hoping he will come back to his own movement which you then, at a later time, work with it again. You go your own way and let the patient go his own way. These things are done in brief moments only, not pursued, and not persisted with.

Many movement therapists do not work this way. They are trying to develop something through a behavioral conditioning approach. This is imposing upon the patient and it will bind him in. As differentiation in movements become more evident you can begin to explore with movement.

You can sometimes put your hands under the patient's hands and let them push your hands down. You are continuing the identification with your body because they have used your hands as part of themselves. Then later begin to work for differentiation between the two bodies. The bodies then begin to become separate and the patient can begin to initiate movement which the therapist can folllow, and the therapist can initiate movements which the patient will follow.

You can sometimes let the patient put his hands under yours and lift your hands so the patient can get a good stretch up. Verbalizing to them, at the same time, that it is easier for them to lift their arms if they lift your arms. The verbalization also helps start an establishment of the differentiation. "The weight of my arms can help you to lift your arms." The reality factor here is that they come to know you know what you are working toward. They become aware you are doing these things for a reason, and they can feel they are "going somewhere" with you, instead of just moving.

Therefore verbalization is used with movements in therapy when the intention in the movement is a positive or definite one. A movement therapist does not cut off from verbalization, she uses it as a tool along with the movement. It helps the patient become aware of why he is moving, aware he is moving with a purpose. Verbalization is not used for "telling" a patient what to do, it is used for helping him know where he is going and why he is going.

When patients understand why they are moving, the reason for the movement, they can get insight into what they are doing.

This does not mean verbalization goes on all the time—only when it is purposeful and has a reason for being.

Regarding being "pulled back" in body movements: The dance therapist would work toward helping the body "come forward" again and be part of the world in an acceptable way to that person. You would use much of the same approach whether the patient was autistic, or schizophrenic. You are trying to get them into the world. Even with a person with angry feelings who carried his body pulled back—because he is afraid of what will happen to the world if he lashes out because it might go beyond his control.

When it is a matter of the body having become pulled back because of the hostility that might come forth the therapist can drive out with shoulders and arms and body, saying "go forward, go forward, go forward". This in turn takes away concentrating on the hostile feelings and works toward moving muscles. The attention is turned to how the body is moving and not necessarily what the movements are symbolizing. This leaves the patient in a safe area for using the same forward movements that they might have used out of control.

This "going forward" use of movement is also done with a depressed person helping him find out it is safe to come out and he won't get hurt. So even with shame of body image rather then with holding back from hostility rhythmic movement can help a person find out he can come out because he won't get hurt and he won't hurt anybody. You do not verbalize it won't hurt them, they just find it out.

After depressed people have used going forward and coming out movements they will begin to ask for these movements. The patients then begin to tell you what it does to them, rather then your telling them. When they can begin to say "I feel uptight" the dance therapist can agree 'Let's get it out". The feeling causing the tightness is not worked with, energy is concentrated on the muscle movement instead. And non-verbally both the patient and the therapist both know the other is aware of the feeling but the action is focused on the use of the muscles.

Space perception and body image:

We are not only in a space outside our body, where space is around us, we are also taking up space, our body is in a space which is filled by the body.

The space or zone immediately around our body is closely interrelated with the body image, acting as a sort of extension of the body.

In pathology, if the patient is very manicy the space around their body is a very wide area. If they are catatonic schizophrenic the space becomes very constricted and is very little beyond their body, if at all. Knowing this the therapist would be very aware of where she could go with his own body before the patient would begin to feel she had intruded into their body image zone. You can move practically on top of a catatonic before he would be aware of you or your body. But his reaction to your closeness can become violent because it is such a supercharged area from being so constricted.

The manic's space is so large and scattered and their body image goes out way beyond them. It is not a nebulous image, but one with tremendous force and feeling of power. The dance thereapist would then use many of the rhythmic movements outside this space zone and have a lot of strong rhythmic action back and forth between herself and the patient, staying far apart, because it will feel "together" with the patient. It becomes a fearful thing if the therapist comes in too close into the patients' extended space.

So you can come closer in movement to a person who is withdrawn than you can to a person who is manic. Although you would be using the same type movements you would use them in a different way. And you would use of lot of ups and downs to the floor keeping your bodies separate when working with a manic patient, letting them go free to encompass the whole room without getting in their way. You would use strong, driving movements with all parts of your body also covering territory with them, but away from them. You would be reflecting the quality of their movements in an effort to establish a relationship with them. You will use closed fists with driving, hostile qualities And when they see you are working with them they can begin to realize these things can be between two people and still be safe. There is no necessity to verbalize this to them.

Body image is created, constructed and developed:

When there is pathology relating to the creation or construction of the body image distortion rather than absence of a body part is the case. The distortion is usually a difference in length, particularly in the leg. There is a feeling of weakness as though the body cannot be supported. This happens with the leg more than other parts of the body.

This doesn't necessarily tie in to whether the person is a manic or schizophrenic, or what, but is an indication that the person is extremely ill.

When these persons are asked to draw a picture of a person. Whatever they draw,whether it is a person or a robot or what, it is usually a reflection of their own body image. And if there is distortion in drawing a picture of a person you usually find that the person's fantasy of what the world is like is also distorted. It reflects a severe illness.

And, conversely, there is the likelihood that if there is a distortion of perception of the outside world, (kinesthetically, tactilly, optically or acoustically) whether from functional or organic causes, you will get a distortion of perception of the body image.

Since motion influences the body image, and a change in the body image leads to a change in the psychic attitude, then if you can work a feeling of distortion of a body image out in motion then this will change your psychic attitude about yourself.

Body image changes constantly:

This changing of body image is enjoyable to a healthy, integrated personality. In pathology the image becomes more inflexible and uptight and not so pleasurable so that you don't feel responsive to change in body size. The body size stays pretty much the same in pathology.

Frequently the person will feel overlarge or inadequate in different aspects of his body image and he stays this way through different experiences rather than "playing around" with his image.

After a body action session, the person who is feeling over-tight, over-large and gross will feel not quite so large. Someone who feels so depressed will feel himself not so inadequate in moving. They become better able to move and change with what they come in contact.

To help the person gain more flexibility the dance therapist would work with contrasting movements such as large movements/small movements; hostile movements/peaceful movements so the patient can feel the difference in the body itself because the muscles are moving. This will eventually, perhaps, hopefully have a reflection on their body image.

The contrasting movements are worked with in a non-threatening way. Working on a mat on the floor is good because it is restful and the person can feel their whole spine, they can feel themselves, their whole body, before they do anything up round the floor. The working on the mat does not change the body image but primarily gets the body feeling movement and stretch and pressure. This then allows the person the mobility with which to make the transition to the floor. They will have relaxed in the joints and in the groups of muscles.

Seeks to gain a "normal" posture:

A person tries to bring his body to a balance a homeostasis. In trying to find it movement is required. There is experimentation in movement. Every postural change brings with it the need to move toward a balance.

In pathology this balance, this "normal" posture, is much more difficult to find. Manics over-react in the search for the normal. Withdrawn persons do not experiment, they like to stay in pacifity, they have fewer postural changes.

In movement therapy you work toward creating postural changes so the patient can experience seeking in a healthy way the "normal" postures for change. With withdrawn persons the therapist might begin body warm-ups with the patient sitting in a chair, then move to the mat, then to the standing position where he can move across the floor, gradually leading the patient into the "more precarious" area for seeking normalcy.

With the person who is scattered and is all over the place the therapist would begin in reverse and bring him in from flights of movement into solid constructs of movement.

You are not working toward re-conditioning of muscular movement as is done in behavioral modification and effort-shape movement. You work toward letting the movements come from the patient so they can experience the feeling. The dance therapist then responds to *that* rather than imposing the muscle movement to condition the postural change. The patient can feel the freedom to try a different number of body postures only when he is ready for it. Only when he is ready for it will it become meaningful to him and effect a change in his body image. His postural movements may change from conditioning but it hasn't necessarily effected a real change within the patient.

It might seem it would take longer to wait and let things happen from within the patient, but this is not necessarily so. And further, when the willingness to experiment with postural changes does come it is of longer duration than from being conditioned and imposed upon. Conditioning stimulates imitation of movement but not "real" movement, it changes the tonic posturing of the muscles and of the body but not the body image.

You can tell a person to raise their arms, but until they feel it inside you won't get the real lift in the body. You can stretch your arms and body up forever and a day and still not feel it inside.

Body image influenced by our perception of gravity and feeling of heaviness as a mass:

Normally we treat our body like any other heavy mass and we perceive the inside of our body as a feeling of emptiness within ourselves.

When there is pathology you often times have very strange feelings within your body. There is a persistence of feeling that your body image shows you have very strange things about your body.

eg. A person can feel an inability to be stretched bilaterally at once because of a feeling of being split down the middle part of the body. There is a fear of being pulled apart if both sides of the body are stretched at the same time out to the sides.

In this case the dance therapist would stretch one arm and one side of the body, then alternate and stretch the other side separately so that the patient wouldn't be "pulled apart".

eg. A person might feel that one leg is shorter than the other, or that the head would fall off if they moved certain ways.

A dance therapist would watch out for all of these things because the distortion is in the patient's positive awareness, and even though it is fantasy it is very real to the patient.

However since we perceive our bodies as empty and a mass, that unless there is specific pain associated with a part of the body, you don't usually have pathology indicated by a change in feeling toward the body mass internally. The distortion is usually external.

Patients do comment about a different weight-feel to parts of their bodies. If they are depressed they sometimes feel their hips are extremely heavy and that their legs are extremely heavy to the point that they move inadequately because they feel they are carrying such weight around with them. They sometimes ask to move sitting in a chair rather than feel the heavy weight of their body on the mat. The chair serves as the support for the weight they do feel rather than their having to depend on supporting themselves. After moving on the chair for a bit they are then able to work on the mat where they still have support and feel safe. This means the dance therapist must take rhythmic movements into the areas where the patient feels best supported. This helps the patient build strength in the back and legs so he will begin to become able to feel he *can* lift his hips and his legs. This also helps the patient feel an increase in mobility from having moved with support first.

As they begin to be limbered up they then begin to feel a normal amount of weight rather than such an excess. And this beginning normal feeling usually carries over from one session to the next, if the sessions are regular. As their body weight begins to feel more normal their depression lifts. And as their depression ends they continue to feel they can move normally, as well as feeling less weighty.

There are persons who do not feel excessive weight but feel an over degree of lightness. This is usually involved with the extremities. The extremities have a feeling of emptiness rather than heavy mass. They feel their arms are so light, or their body is so light, that it will break apart. The normal weight-feel we have to help locate ourselves leaves these patients and they feel they can't risk moving their head or whatever, or risk stretching out or they might split more.

It is usually the schizophrenic who feels this kind of lightness and is deep in a fantasy world. So depression usually comes with heavy weight feeling, a schizophrenic usually feels weightless and as though he will dissolve into mid-air. This is why they seem less able to know where they are in space.

The primary sensations of body image come from special configuration of stimuli on the skin

By touching or rubbing the skin or by moving our muscles which stimulate the skin we delineate the surface of our bodies.

Some patients will rub their hands or arms repeatedly (or other parts of their bodies). It seems to give them a sense of unity, of surface delineation. The dance therapist will take these movements and put them into rhythmic action to work toward helping the patient find himself in space. It's a search for "where am I?"

By having the patient rub his hands against his thighs it can sometimes help him become better able to put his legs into motion.

Patients who wring their hands are many times trying to get rid of something, it is as if he is rubbing guilt off trying to get a clear feeling of his body again as uncontaminated. This is also true of wringing ones hands in grief. The person is trying to get rid of the tension of guilt—of the guilt feelings one may have had against the person for whom one is grieving.

The dance therapist would take the hand-wringing movements into rhythmic action to get them more open; many times working on into "throwing-away" movements in various directions—over the shoulder—saying non-verbally "Let's get rid of it."

Since the sensations just below the surface of the skin are the primary source of body image the dance therapist uses the muscles to stimulate the areas under the surface of the skin. This helps the person to begin to feel "warmed up" and more aware of the area of the body with which they are working. This helps them find where their body is.

All of therapeutic body movement is geared toward getting in touch with as much of the skin surface as you can—whether you are using body postures of sitting and touching walking and lying down to feel the pressure on the skin; you use the muscles to stimulate the skin over the different parts of the body from within.

You are working on actions that are intangible, that cannot be demonstrated because they belong to the feeling tone of the individual that will not always come forth at the time of a session. This is the difference between behavioral conditioning and effort shape movements which are working with tangible forms of movements and are looking for tangible results in regard to the way the patient moves. When working with dance therapy and feeling tones of the patients the patients show you the feeling tone when and if they are ready and they may never verbalize about it. And there is no way to put this feeling tone into the patient with tangible and manipulative type movements that are labeled.

Body image is inseparably involved with emotions and action:

When the emotions become pathologically oriented then the body stays in that pathological area of action, and the body image becomes distorted.

The dance therapist works with the essentially healthy aspects of the emotions and hopefully these healthy aspects will have a reflection in the body action and eventually in the body image.

Fear is normal but continuing fear is pathological, passing fear is a normal reaction. If the patient is withdrawn from continuing fear and the therapist can work with an outgoing type of motion, this will perhaps reduce the degree of fixation of fear because the patient hasn't stayed in an action position of fear but is moving in action expressing non-fear.

When there is an anger fixation the therapist uses the movement expressions of force—movements reflecting driving force of hostile movements, which will then relax the person and then reduce the need for feeling this hostility as an outgoing thing.

The dance therapist uses the emotions in actions in such a way that there are no destructive consequences from having expressed the emotions which can help the patient drop the degree of pathological fixation on the emotion. The patient has been able to use the action of the emotions in ways that has hurt no one, has relaxed the patient, and has not even hurt himself.

And basically it is the rhythmic quality of the expression which makes this possible. Simply using the aggressive movements per se does not help that much. Mere expression of the emotion with action does not change the body image. The body image begins to change in response to the rhythmic action, because you are forced to be more aware of your body moving at a time you want it to move under the control of the patient rather than the emotion. Through the non-verbal communication and interrelationship going on during the rhythmic action both the patient and the therapist are aware of the implications of the movements, but because there is an understanding that they both know what could happen with the movements and because they are both working with the rhythm in the movement there is no need felt for the movement to be realized in its destructive form. Patients have expressed their awareness verbally after the dance therapy sessions.

The patients are also receiving a simultaneous non-verbal message from the therapist that she accepts the feeling behind the movement and understands, is not afraid of it and works basically on seeing how she and the patient can use the movement together in a way that is accepted. It becomes a shared experience, which then drops away the destructive aspects of the movement. The relationship between the patient and the therapist becomes the paramount thing, because they are relating to the rhythmic quality of the movement that is outside both of themselves. They are sharing the action and not the destructiveness of the action.

This leaves the patient free to go on to other things because they have released for the moment the pathological fixation. And this happens without having to verbalize what is going on. The emotion is recognized without having to have been openly confronted to it.

Hostile patients particularly will many times dance "against" the dance therapist and then return to be able to dance "with" her because of the change that takes place within themselves. They will at times verbalize for themselves that now that they have danced against you they can dance with you.

Tension and relaxation of muscles are elementary components in the dynamic sequence of displaying energy and losing energy. There is a close interrelationship between this muscular sequence and the psychic attitude of the person. Every sequence of tension and relaxation provokes a specific attitude.

This is why a dance therapist will use stretches, and the pulling of the body apart, and then the relaxing. It will begin to help the patient feel more alive. It's a natural sequence for feeling more alive. And this changes his attitude about himself. It changes the inner situation and atttitudes and even provokes a fantasy situation which fits the muscular sequence. The person feels more vital.

And by working with the psycho-motor disturbance and changing its action into a different motor action one can "come down" or "come up" from a particular emotional state into a different emotion *and* attitude.

Body image formation is primarily a social creation:

Usually the attitude toward different parts of one's body can be determined by the interest the persons around us give to our body.

But when there is pathology it doesn't matter what somebody else is thinking, because the person has the peculiar ideas about himself. This is when body image construction, as a result of attitudes of others, becomes irrelevant because the patient has become so deeply involved in his own pathology that he determines these things about his body, and withdraws from social influence even though it has perhaps been negative social influence which originated his pathology.

This is where dance therapy can come in with helping reestablish the influence on the patient of the attitudes of other people around him. Identification with the therapist or the group movement leader through the rhythmic movements can often bring back social awareness and acceptance of social influence.

In the therapy, whatever is coming across through rhythmic movement can affect the patient's body image, just as this is done in social relationships in general. We have a normal tendency to elaborate our body image according to the experiences we obtain through the actions and attitudes of others.

Dance therapy is a key area where body images can be recreated and constructed because there is so much action and the relationship between the therapist and the patient (and other patients in the group) *is* social. There is a merging and a separating of identification of body images as people move together rhythmically.

In normal persons one's own body image and the body image of others are not primarily dependent upon each other—they are equal and independent of each other. In pathology the ill person's body image is dependent upon the other person. Many times the patient will say for the dance therapist to move against him more heavily so he can know where the dance therapist is and thus know where he is. This is because the patient has negated so much that comes from within himself whereas a healthy person has much that does come from within himself with which to construct his own body image in a realistic and healthy way. It is through this temporary dependency on the body of the therapist that the patient can come back and be able to use his own body to create his own body image.

Where in normal circumstances a body is a body among other bodies, a person with pathology cuts this off and withdraws and thus begin a pathological cycle:

Loss of relationship with the outside world = loss of interest in the creating and continual construction of ones own body = loss of awareness of oneself as a personality = depersonalization = loss of relationship with the outside world.

This is why it is preferable in dance therapy to work with more than one person. It is better to have other people there as well as the therapist so there can be others to relate to as well. This reduces a one-to-one identification and increases to the opportunity for the patient to become involved in creating and constructing his own body image rather than staying dependent upon the therapist. Interest in oneself and interest in others runs parallel.

PART V

About

Three selections about Marian Chace are included to give balance and perspective. One by Edith M. Stern presents the human side of Marian; a second by Irmgard Bartenieff gives an analytic assessment of Marian's stature as a major figure in the development of dance therapy; Eithne Tabor's poem speaks for itself.

She Breaks Through Invisible Walls

Reprinted courtesy of the National Association for Mental Health, Inc., from *Mental Hygiene*, 41 (July, 1957), pp. 363-371.

EDITH M. STERN *

With a portable victrola and a touch of the hand a dancer named Marian Chace has started thousands of mental patients on the road to recovery. Going along with her day after day as she did her healing work at St. Elizabeths Hospital, Washington, D.C., I saw seeming miracles occur. Women, rigid and remote in catatonic stupor, began to move again and even faintly to smile. Angry manics, shouting imprecations and obscenities at their "voices," their attendants and their fellow-patients when we came in, quieted down within a very few minutes, stopped their restless pacing and sudden aimless darting across the floor and joined in group relaxing exercises. Zombie-like men, who for years had failed to respond to all other forms of treatment and were sunk deep in silence and apathy, one by one rose from the benches on which they were listlessly sitting or lying and came alive, tossing a ball to music, talking and rhythmically swinging their arms and legs.

Marian Chace's way with mental patients, like that of anyone successful in helping them, is partly an intangible matter of personality. Radiant and relaxed, gracious and mature, she emanates sensitivity and understanding. But fortunately the crux of her spectacular ability to reach the unreachable, to win over the hostile, to strike the spark of life again in the living dead, to reassure those so hurt and frightened by reality that they dare not let themselves move or speak, is both specific and imitable. To break through the invisible walls with which all psychotics surround themselves to keep people away, she uses primitive means of communication that go deeper than words—rhythm, movement and touch. Old and fundamental as humanity itself, simple and universal as mothers' crooning and rocking their babies in their arms, these catch patients off guard, painlessly crumble their defenses, make them more receptive to other approaches. Over and over again she demonstrates that there is more strength in the mentally ill than most of us realize, and that they can use it if we do not frighten them.

I went with Marian Chace to a locked ward of disturbed women, most of them just admitted. "I have no idea what we'll run into," she told me

Mrs. Stern is well known for her popular magazine articles and books on aspects of mental illness and health. A new edition of her widely-read *Mental Illness–A Guide for the Family*, originally published in 1942, appears on Harper & Brothers' current list.

beforehand. "So you'd better leave your eyeglasses and earrings in my office. These patients are about as sick as anyone can get; they're quarrelsome and assaultive, and their movements are quick and unpredictable."

But I didn't have a bit of trouble during the hour and a half I sat beside the victrola. Let a woman approach me loweringly or suspiciously, all I had to do was to smile and say, "I'm a friend of Miss Chace's," and she would drift quietly away. Via a few old-timers on the ward, and the hospital grapevine, Miss Chace explained to me later, word had got round that she was a "safe" person who didn't intrude, didn't demand anything of you. "I simply create an atmosphere in which they are free to dance—if and as they wish," she says.

Nothing could have been less like the usual dancing class than the session of dance therapy. There was no attempt to teach steps or skills, only suggestions to make simple movements possible for anyone—shaking wrists, or swinging legs, or rolling hips. No formation lasted more than a few minutes, for these excitable patients have no longer concentration span than a three-year-old. Sometimes a dozen women, sometimes only three or four, moved rhythmically together in a circle. Some twirled and whirled all by themselves, or with imaginary partners, outside the circles. At times there were dancing pairs. A pale thin girl with agonized eyes turned a chair towards the wall and sat in it with her back to the moving figures during most of the session; then suddenly she jumped up and bending and leaping to calypso music joined the others. Shortly before we left, a white-capped attendant came in with a fresh supply of towels; spontaneously and lithely she fell into lively stepping; a patient put an arm around her waist and the two of them danced merrily away together. It was all only a little mad, and very gay. No one got into a fight, although the number of women in felt slippers and one with patches on her face evidenced kicking and scratching could be anticipated. Not once did I hear the screams or tirades or shrill conversations with voices typical on such wards. The only loud sounds were the laughter of women who seemed to be thoroughly enjoying themselves.

On the surface, the session seemed like merely free-for-all activity, apparently aimless recreation. But important things had happened to troubled minds. Through moving to music—"And that's all dancing is," says Marian Chace—the patients had healthfully released sick anger and hatreds.

One heavy-set middle-aged woman, for instance, who did nothing but pace during the beginning of the session started vigorous bending movements in time to a lusty tune.

"Scrub, scrub, scrub," she chanted.

Marian Chace made similar movements alongside her, and chimed in with "Scrub, scrub, scrub" too.

Continuing her rhythmic bending from the waist, the woman held out her arms and simultaneously took big forward strides. Again Miss Chace, beside her, adapted her pantomine. "Scrub, scrub, scrub, and pushing a baby carriage," the woman remarked. "You can do it at the same time."

Next she moved her arms round and round. "Sometimes you stir the food," she said. Then suddenly she urged, "Put your head on my shoulder."

Marian Chace did so. The patient put her head on Miss Chace's shoulder and grasping her around the waist held her close. Responsively Miss Chace put her arm around the patient's waist and the two of them moved up and down together, up and down, each time going lower with each downward dip until they were nearly lying on the floor. For a moment I was terrified; I thought that the large, irresponsible former housewife was going to choke the dance therapist. But thc minute the music stopped she broke her hold, stood up very straight and tall, grinned broadly and exclaimed, "Golly, isn't that a relief!" Indeed, her mood remained so amiable that she escorted us to the end of the corridor as we were leaving and, turning to me, graciously complimented me on being such a beautiful dancer—although I hadn't left my chair.

Later Miss Chace interpreted for me what had happened. "She was acting out her hatred of domestic drudgery. When she said 'Isn't that a relief!' she meant that she had been close to someone who understands her problems and feels as she does. A few times more of releasing through body-action the feelings she's still too sick to put into words, of wordless assurance that she has a congenial friend, and she'll be accessible to verbal psychotherapy with her doctor."

On wards where men or women are depressed and withdrawn, too quiet rather than too active, there is little similar, spontaneous plunging into expressive movement. Here Miss Chace has to draw out, woo, induce participation in even such simple activities as taking slow easy rhythmic steps. But wherever she holds the dance sessions she uses the sequence of rhythm, movement and touch.

On a ward of depressed women, sitting with their eyes fixed on nowhere, standing still and stiff against the wall or crouching dismally on the floor in doorways, as far away as they could get from everyone else on the ward, the first records Marian Chace plays are attuned to the prevailing sad slow mood. Then she begins to circulate about the day-room, gracefully undulating, swaying, as she approaches one silent sick individual after another. With a warm, gentle "Won't you dance with us? We need you," or wordlessly, she holds out her arms, not high, so they do not seem threatening. I saw woman after woman begin stiffly and tentatively to move rhythmically too, then put out her hands and timorously, slowly place them in the dance therapist's.

As a step toward recovery a mental patient's willingness to hold hands can be as momentous as a baby's first word in the process of growing up. "Psychotics don't want to be touched" is a truism in mental hospitals. "I never take patients' hands," says Marian Chace. "I let them take mine, when they are ready through their response to music and movement."

And she can tell when they are ready, she maintains, not through second sight nor some mysterious kind of intuition, but because of her training as a dancer. As all of us can judge roughly the way normal people feel through their facial expressions or tone of voice, so she can gauge to a find point whether or not patients want to make contact with her by their bodies, by the way they sit or stand, pull back a little or lean slightly forward, whether their muscles are tense or relaxed.

Observing her at work, questioning her, learning from her, with her permission I tried out for myself some of her wordless technique of invisible wall break-through. The first time, on a men's ward, I started out all right but then made a mistake. I managed to draw into the dancing a middle-aged man, very busy shaking his fist at his voices and moving his lips silently at them. I had swayed before him, a little distance away, holding out my hands in wordless invitation. The fist opened and he placed his right hand in mine. Then his left hand which had been up in the air, moved slowly down to my shoulder. I neither drew back nor moved forward, thus communicating—as I had learned from Miss Chace one must—that I was neither fearful nor trying to impose myself on him. Apparently he felt safe, for his other hand moved into mine too, and I had a moment of triumph when we did some simple steps together. But it did not last long. All of a sudden the hands pulled away, not angrily, only in a gesture of "Leave me alone now, I've had enough," and he returned to acting on his delusions.

"What did I do wrong? What would you have done?" I asked Miss Chace later.

"From reading and experience I'd have known he was too sick to sustain any but the briefest contact," she said, "but even if I hadn't I could have told by the tension of his handclasp when it was time to leave him before he left me."

Next time, on a woman's ward, I was able to do better. The patient was an angry-looking woman who when we entered was cursing and shouting furiously, "They've been sticking pins in my behind!"

Marian Chace promptly adapted her mood. "Well," she said indignantly, standing hand on hips, belligerently before the patient, "that's what they did to you, did they!"

Somewhat mollified by this evidence of fellow-feeling, the patient retorted a bit less angrily, "They sure did!"

"Well, it must have been good for you, or they wouldn't have," Marian Chace continued casually, "and dancing will be good for you too, so won't you do it with us?"

Without another word the woman arose, put her hands in Marian Chace's and started a stately minuet-type dance. Freeing Miss Chace to get in other dancers, I took her over. I had learned that one does not attempt to determine the type of dancing; one goes along with what the patient indicates. So we held our clasped hands high, pirouetted gravely and made deep curtsies to each other like two grand ladies. Dignified, and wordlessly accorded dignity, the patient's hostile expression changed to one of serene and lofty satisfaction, and everything seemed to be going fine until I felt her hand begin to tighten around my wrist. I dropped it promptly, leaving her free to go stepping off by herself, and we therefore remained friends. Much later in the session, in the midst of releasing anger by banging the palms of her hands savagely on the floor in time to lively music, she paused for a moment to give me a good-natured wink.

The first few patients are the hardest to get started. As the sessions go on a kind of contagion develops, and more and more join in unasked. Miss Chace bides her time with those who remain aloof through two, three or more sessions; she never urges, is never importunate, never puts anyone in the position of seeming to turn her down. In this permissive atmosphere, a softening-up occurs even in those most fearful, most locked-in, most suspicious. One old lady after weeks of silent watching, finally entered the hand-holding circle. "I'm glad you're with us," Marian Chace welcomed her. "Why, Miss Chace," the old lady answered reproachfully, "I've been with you all the time!'

The difference between two sessions on the same ward, a week apart, was amazing. At the first, only about a dozen danced at all, never more than three or four together. At the second, not only were there more than twice as many participants, but a group spirit had been born. The patients were clearly more aware of one another, at times reaching for each other's hands, getting hangers-back into the circle.

I attended a dance session for women with whom Miss Chace had worked more frequently. There I had the sense of a group which had really jelled. Most of the women danced as if they felt common aims and interests and companionship.

Many of this "Dance Group," as by their own wish they are known, are young schizophrenics who realize that they are maladjusted, consciously want help, but can't take straight, super-imposed advice. They tend to talk in a roundabout way rather than directly, in poetic symbols rather than in facts. For instance, to convey that she is troubled, a girl may say, "I'm in a boat, rocking in rough water" or she is disastrously inhibited, "You can learn a lot from babies—they're all exposed; they don't hold anything within themselves." With indirection similar to theirs Miss Chace uses words as a supplement to body action.

For instance, when she wanted the group to realize that they had mastery over their bodies, would feel more self-confident if they acted more self-confident, she played a tango record and told how Argentinian girls are taught to stand straight and proud. "Now let's be like Argentinians," she suggested. Hunched shoulders straightened, dejected heads went high, as the women adlibbed to the music. "Humph," one of them remarked, "we're from a depressed and suicidal ward, but we certainly don't look it now, do we?"

To a stimulating tune Miss Chace said, "Make your hands into fists and then let go!" Most in the circle hit out energetically at an invisible antagonist, but to one, moving her arms inwards, she commented smilingly, "Why beat yourself?" And she subtly gave insight into other unuttered feelings through a neck-bending exercise. "Way back," she urged. "Oh, way back! Fine! Some people are afraid to put their necks back—they feel vulnerable." Another dance movement, to a waltz, involved wide sweeps of the arms. "Take love into yourself," said Miss Chace, dancing as if she were doing exactly that, "then you can give it out again."

She continually encourages the group to make its own interpretations of bodily motions with such questions as "What does this remind you of?" or "What shall we do now?" "Walk through a large room, to people you like and who like you," a slender blonde proposed. "All right, go towards those friendly people," Miss Chace took her up. "Walk not thinking of yourself but of them. That's it! Good! Funny how differently you move when you really want to get somewhere, isn't it?"

Out of the Dance Group has developed group dramatics. The patients always determined their own dance activities, like parties or decorating the dance room. But even so in the spring of 1954 Miss Chace was somewhat startled, after having been away two weeks, to be greeted with a new kind of request.

"We want to do a show about a group of women living together and the funny and painful things that happen to them," the girl acting as spokesman for the group announced. "Since we're all living together in a mental hospital, we want to do it about that. We can dream too, and we do—and since our dreams include men, of course, may we invite them to join us?"

The outcome was a patient-written, patient-produced and patient-acted satire with music and dancing, "Hotel St. Elizabeths." It had five pairs of scenes, the first showing the realities of hospital life, like the lack of privacy in a dormitory, the second wishful thinking—a luxurious boudoir, complete with lady's maid and lover. Popular songs were parodied:

"I hear voices and there's no one there
I see visions floating in the air
I have nightmares in the daylight glare

I wonder why, I wonder why.
Schizophrenia is new to me,
I'm a double personality
Doctors say one's enough for me,
I wonder why, I wonder why."

and "We are poor little girls with our minds awry."

The group did its own encouraging. One woman, with consummate patience, taught an awkward man to tango with her. It also did its own disciplining. The group won over and toned down a difficult male patient who had been ejected from every hospital recreational activity; he always wanted to be the whole show and in the band, for example, had insisted on playing so loud that he drowned out everyone else.

Other patients besides the cast took part in the production. One girl who had sat aloof at rehearsals after two weeks offered to be script girl and made many helpful suggestions. Old ladies on geriatric wards made leis for a Hawaiian scene; costumes were sewed in the occupational therapy workshop. Altogether, so successful and therapeutic was the project that the hospital administration requested the Dance Group to create a pageant on the life of Dorothea Lynde Dix, St. Elizabeths founder, for the centennial celebration in May 1955.

For months beforehand the St. Elizabeths Players—as the Dance Group now chose to call itself—worked, together with many other patients from various wards, on an ambitious production, "Cry of Humanity." Part play, part pageant, part ballet, running three hours, it held successive audiences of invited distinguished guests, patients, patients' relatives, the Mental Hospital Institute and the general public spellbound. Moving, remarkably dramatic and finished, it portrayed patients' own interpretation of Dorothea Dix's life and works and the problems of the mentally ill. They themselves, under Marian Chace's direction, did the research, wrote the script, structured the ballets. They chose the cast, after try-outs; they made the scenery and costumes; they scrubbed the stage.

Some of the cast were under indictments. Some, when they were off-stage, conversed volubly with their voices. Few were allowed to go about unattended. Old-timers from a male chronic ward formed a chorus. The cast was constantly in flux as substitutions were made for those who left the hospital to go home. Yet through the whole long period of preparation and seven performances, I was told, there was less bickering, fewer emotional upsets or untoward incidents, than in the course of the usual amateur show.

On May 15, 1955 scenes from "Cry of Humanity" were televised from film on the March of Medicine program. One was Dorothea Dix's visit to the jail where she first saw demented, half-clad, half-starved women kept in cages like wild animals; with chilling realism 20th century patients enacted what they would have been in the 19th. One was a ballet of her dreams, another her impassioned plea to the Massachusetts legislators. During the shooting the patients' endurance and composure never flagged for long, grueling days. Over and over they had to be under blinding lights, repeat the same lines, keep quiet when necessary. This self-control, this working together for a common end, came from people so turned in on themselves, so unable to give and take, that they needed care in a mental hospital!

"And it all grew out of dancing," says Marian Chace. Other patient-conceived and created dramatic and dance productions, under her direction, followed "Cry of Humanity." "The Skitsofrolics" was a satire on various phases of hospital treatment. In "Free Horizons," first presented May 1, 1957, the theme of mental illness was broadened to that of loneliness in the outside world; the protagonist is a Hungarian seeking the place in the United States where he will find himself at home. After this, Miss Chace says frankly, she does ot know what the patients will develop as they literally move towards health.

Indeed her whole life has been a progression of one thing leading to the larger next. A successful concert dancer and choreographer, she never expected to be a full-fledged staff member of a mental hospital's psychotherapy branch.

Marian Chace was born in Providence, R. I., in 1896, of an old family with intellectual and Puritan traditions. She attended Brown University, then moved with her family to Washington. There she met and fell in love with a handsome young dancer named Lester Shafer, who urged her to study where he did, at the Denishawn School in New York. Ruth St. Denis and her husband, Ted Shawn, its directors, taught all forms of the dance except tap and ballroom, and the school was ascetically dedicated to the art of the dance. Students had to eat frugally, keep regular hours, were not allowed to smoke or drink.

Marian loved to dance and together with Shafer to create dance forms. Offered a vaudeville tour, they decided to make it a wedding trip and then settled in Los Angeles, where their golden-haired daughter was born. Six weeks later Marian was dancing again, and soon afterwards she and her husband went on tour with the Denishawn dancers as part of the Ziegfeld Follies. Beautiful, and wearing costumes well, Marian served as a show girl besides dancing with the Denishawn troupe. Even after the couple had opened a Denishawn branch in Washington, she remained a performer, a creator of dance arrangements, rather than a teacher. She taught primarily to develop skilled dancers—some of whom went on to Broadway—to dance before large audiences with her.

Many students continued to come for lessons, however, who lacked the stuff to become artists, would never make the grade as professional dancers, and knew it. She began to wonder why. What satisfaction did they get from dancing? In 1938 she got an inkling of the answer. Shafer and she had been separated; she was continuing the school alone and was engaged, as a kind of frill, to give weekly dancing lessons to children in a Maryland boarding school. Most of the youngsters were from broken homes; they were upset, maladjusted, obstreperous. Miss Chace noted that hair-pullings, crying and rudeness stopped almost miraculously during group dancing; that often the most rebellious child, feeling he had a part to play, had leadership qualities before used only for mischief-making. Interest in the emotional values of dancing led her to volunteer the next summer at the National Training School for Girls, the next at an orphanage.

Nevertheless others recognized her unique therapeutic skill before she realized it herself. Her school began to be known as a place where you could dance away difficulties. Pediatricians and orthopedists whose own little girls had been in her beginners' classes sent small patients to become better adjusted emotionally, to improve in coordination. Jittery government workers attended evening classes to relax and gain self-confidence. A lawyer danced himself out of stuttering. In 1939-40 Miss Chace was asked to conduct a seminar for D. C. teachers of exceptional children.

Her move to St. Elizabeths in 1942 was almost a happy accident. "I think you'd be wonderful with mental patients," said the mother of one of her child-pupils. "Have you ever worked with them?" Marian Chace said no, but she'd love to try.

She began as a part-time volunteer with the Red Cross. Very quickly she had such astounding results with patients that she was spotted as providing not merely recreation but a true though unorthodox form of psychotherapy, and in 1944 she was asked to come full-time on the Red Cross payroll. Giving up her school with a pang, except for one advanced class which she retains to this day, she devoted herself to psychoneurotic veterans. In 1947 Red Cross funds were cut off. But Dr. Winfred Overholser, St. Elizabeths progressive superintendent, wasn't going to let Miss Chace go. He transferred her to the regular staff payroll.

Neither Dr. Overholser nor anyone else could tell me how many of the hundreds of men and women who after an average stay of less than a year and a half leave St. Elizabeths each year to live again in the community owe their discharge directly to Miss Chace. St. Elizabeths affords many other treatments besides dance therapy—among them drugs, verbal group psychotherapy, occupational and recreational therapy, hydrotherapy—and it is impossible to evaluate the contribution of each. "But I *can* say this," Dr. Overholser declared. "Marian Chace has made the initial dent in many, some of them resistive to all other forms of treatment."

Today at St. Elizabeths dance therapy is one of the first activities offered to new patients, and with the psychiatrists Marian Chace participates in staff conferences. Since she has been at St. Elizabeths she has studied at the Washington School of Psychiatry. She teaches nurses, psychologists, student nurses and student chaplains as part of the hospital's training program.

Many other mental hospitals—state, private and VA—have invited her to demonstrate for them. She has taken part in numerous national psychiatric and music therapists' conferences, has spoken on dance therapy before audiences with strings of degrees, written on "non-verbal communication" in learned journals.

Others, says Miss Chace, can learn to do dance therapy; women who have trained with her have already launched it in state hospitals in Iowa and Colorado, at the VA Hospital in Battle Creek, Mich. One must, in the first place, be a dancer; otherwise, on the one hand patients will react adversely to the therapist's lack of bodily control, of flexibility, of balance, of easy movement, and on the other the therapist will be unable fully to recognize the significance of their movements, detect slight, unobvious muscular tensions. Second, one must really like people and accept them as they are, meet them always with respect as equals.

But even without the services of a real dance therapist, she says, tens of thousands of patients now deteriorating in wretched idleness in mental hosptals all over the United States would benefit by regular dance periods arranged by nurses and attendants. All they need to do is to play dance music, indicate their own readiness to dance, and let the patients engage in free movement for a little while to feel joy and peace.

In fact, Marian Chace believes from the bottom of her heart and experience, we'd all do well to get over the repressions, the inhibitions, the self-consciousness which our civilization has put on the impulse to make rhythmic movements, to dance. "Why does practically everyone look sheepish when I ask, 'Do you ever turn on the radio or phonograph and dance when you're all by yourself?' " she says with a twinkle in her eye. "After all, our most easily available, least expensive, freest means of healthful self-expression and emotional release are our own bodies."

Dance Therapy: A New Profession or a Rediscovery of an Ancient Role of the Dance?

Reprinted courtesy of the American Dance Guild from *Dance Scope*, 7 (Fall-Winter, 1972-1973), pp. 6-18.

IRMGARD BARTENIEFF *

Dance therapy seems all of a sudden to have become an issue, a subject of concern, dispute, and curiosity in the dance world itself. Actually this is not an astonishing development. Those of us working in the field who have our roots in the dance world of the thirties and forties—or even farther back—see it as a direct outgrowth of modern dance, with its rebellious philosophy, here and in Europe. The modern dancer broke with fading art concepts, with the frozen modes of expression in the highly mannered art of Western ballet of the eighteenth and nineteenth centuries, its emphasis on the theatrical and its near absolute formality of structure. The rebellion of modern dance also directed itself against the romantic-idealizations of the fairytale princess-prince romance and the superhuman, ethereal, elusive, doll-like role of the classical ballerina.

Modern dance replaced the fading content of Western dance with certain key notions: spontaneity, authenticity of individual expression, awareness of the body, themes that stressed a whole range of feelings and relationships. The great pioneers of its early years personified themes of human conflict, despair, frustration, and social crisis. Frequently the choreography of the modern dancer crystallized into the age-old form of ritual. Such key innovations lead directly to the essence of dance therapy.

It seems particularly timely to speak at this moment to the dancer about dance therapy, for dance therapy finds itself, after a period of pioneering initiated by outstanding dance personalities, in a new stage of rapid expansion, great diversity, and growth in numbers of practitioners and agencies that seek their services. At the same time we are witnessing a new phase in modern dance, a new era of experimentation that shows marked shifts in forms toward the psychological, the absurd, and toward a sort of borderline theatre with an open stage and participating audiences. Furthermore, what has been developing in dance education, particularly in work with children, resembles the area of the dance therapist even closer and actually overlaps with it in theories of child development.

The key notions of modern dance are clearly reflected in the pioneers of

A former student of Rudolf von Laban and a dancer who had her own troupe in Europe, Irmgard Bartenieff, after coming to the United States published the first work in this country on Labanotation. She was a co-founder of the Dance Notation Bureau, where she now heads the Effort/Shape program, and has also worked for nearly two decades with the physically handicapped and emotionally disturbed.

dance therapy. Starting in the forties and early fifties, these innovators set the stage and models for the present generation of dance therapists, each in a highly individualistic way. They stimulated the development of a number of different approaches now in use. But the starting point and roots of their work remained in dance. I will name five here: Franziska Boas, Marian Chace, Lilyan Espenak on the East coast, and Trudi Schoop and Mary Whitehouse on the West Coast. These five were modern dancers of different background and personality who set the precedents for dance therapy. Not specific "training" but a set of circumstances for each of them led to fateful encounters with the area of mental illness, psychiatry, and psychoanalysis whereby they "discovered" dance as a therapeutic tool in the rehabilitation or, rather, reorganization of disturbed behavior.

Franziska Boas, in 1941, became involved in an experiment with disturbed children under twelve years of age. It was initiated by a personal friend, Dr. Laretta Bender, then a child psychiatrist at Bellevue Hospital, in New York City. She commented afterward in an article written with Dr. Bender on the influence of modern dance techniques in their work. She enumerated some of these elements: use of primitive posture change, like rolling on the floor, crawling; large motor movements; walking and jumping, supported and stimulated by rhythmical accompaniment—essentially percussion—in conjunction with creative use of role-playing, such as, of animals, leaders, commanders. These activities elicited talk from either regressed mute or kinetically hyperactive children. The children talked about their fantasies in playing these roles which provided release of tensions and feeling, and thus supplied direct, authentic information to the psychiatrist.

Marian Chace emerged from the Denishawn group as a concert dancer. She started work with hyperactive and otherwise emotionally disturbed children in her dance studio. Through the parents of these children and their psychotherapists she first entered St. Elizabeth Hospital, in Washington, D.C., as a volunteer. She then established herself as a fulltime therapist and devoted many years to working with many types of hospitalized and discharged mental patients. In her writing she stresses again and again that dance is communication of feeling. She sees the therapist's role as stimulating interaction, as an empathetic catalyst in the process of reintegrating body and mind. She worked in large and small groups, picking up movement utterances of individual patients. This would develop into a movement dialogue by enlarging or transforming the movement theme. In this process the patient began to experience a transformation and liberation from some of his destructiveness or alienation, thus opening channels of communication for the regressed, bodily frozen patient. Being able to have dialogue with the therapist was frequently also the first step toward becoming a member of the group.

Talking while dancing, Chace elicited the verbalizing of feelings, thus readying the patient for other forms of therapeutic intervention. Her work made her a close associate of members of the medical staff and created a relationship of mutual respect. Her understanding and cooperation with psychologists and psychiatrists enabled her to develop over the years a set of professional standards by which to train and guide young dance therapists. Her standards called for responsibility, integrity, and devotion to the patient, as well as constant growth and personal development. At all times, though, she stayed within the realm of dance. Throughout her time at St. Elizabeth she involved larger and smaller groups of patients in dance and music productions that were entirely written, rehearsed, and put together by patients, with music and dance therapists acting in the capacity of consultants. Involvement in the responsibilities of such a cooperative task in many cases would be an indication of the patient's ability to function in a community. Chace later also included psychodrama in her work. She was able to transfer to and impress upon her students her specific kind of understanding and cooperating with psychologists and psychiatrists. She never crossed the dangerous line to pseudopsychiatric authority. The definite role and clear identification she gave the dance therapist, which differed from other therapists—occupational or physical—made her the driving force in the founding of the American Dance Therapy Association (ADTA), in 1965-66, when she gathered together not only her own students but a group of dance-trained people who were working as dance therapists from a variety of approaches.

Lilyan Espenak came to the United States with a European modern dance background and here became associated with a group of Adlerian psychotherapists. This led her to use her extensive experience in teaching dance in therapeutic work with neurotic and psychotic patients and also in work with retarded and mentally defective children. Through her affiliation with New York Medical College (Flower Fifth Hospital), she developed the first extensive training programs (eight months' long) for dance therapists. Her work stresses reintegration of posture as an integral part or the base for developing or reintegrating the body-mind problems of the patients. She also makes use of the whole arsenal of the modern dance educator: music, improvisation, and props, such as, masks, fans, percussion instruments. For a number of years she has worked in close professional contact with the bioenergetic group of Dr. Alexander Lowen, which I will discuss later.

On the West coast about the same time as in the East, two dance personalities developed dance therapy approaches in their own highly individual work.

Trudi Schoop, who is Swiss born, was known to European dance audiences as the pantomimist who created the delightful, endearing, innocent, mischievous Fridolin, the central character of a number of ballets in which she toured. In a curious twist of fate, her first encounter with hospitalized mental patients came just with the trouble-filled times of the early Nazi regime and the threat of impending war. After her Swiss dance group was dissolved, she settled in California and began to work with hospitalized and neurotic patients in close collaboration with psychiatrists. In one of the ADTA Newsletters she summarizes the underlying philosophy of her work and of dance therapy in general:

> If I am correct in assuming that mind and body are interactive, I feel a problem of mental disturbance can be influenced from either side. When psychoanalysis brings about a change in the mental attitude, there should be a corresponding physical change. And when dance therapy brings about a change in the body behavior, there should be a corresponding change in the mind. The approach to verbal therapy is through mind-body. The approach of dance therapy is through body-mind. Both methods want to change the total being, mind and body.

(The first full presentation of her work and philosophy is about to be published in a book under the title *Lost Paradise*.)

Mary Whitehouse emerged from a partly American, partly European modern dance experience and training. Her approach to what she calls "movement" therapy developed from this dance background and from her personal contact with Jungian psychoanalysis. The two became tightly interwoven: She emphasizes that the origin of authentic or true or spontaneous movement response arises from body awareness—an awareness of inner impulse and readiness to move. Making symbolic representation of inner experiences through movement, particularly of dream life, while trying to link these experiences verbally, shows the Jungian influence on her body-mind concept as an inescapable whole. Sensation, emotion, imagination are one in dance-movement action.

A common thread runs through the work of these pioneers of dance therapy, as well as through their philosophy. These five, so different in background, personality, and life experience, share a deep commitment to the life-asserting elements of the dance and to its ability to heighten body-mind awareness, to renew the feeing of wholeness, through rhythmic action to evoke feeling and transform it and represent it in direct and symbolized ways, and through the interaction of dancing in a group to socialize and order human relationships. It seems to this author that the particular sensitivity to these elemental qualities was intensified and deepened as each was affected by the upheavals of the late thirties and the war years that followed. Each of them underwent a crucial process of inner transformation in which communication with an audience from the stage became direct exchange with the person to be helped. It is the return to the old, old role of community healer. All, in their individual language, were to decribe to their students as an essential prerequisite for becoming dance therapists the process of change from performing artist into empathetic catalyst—Marian Chace particularly constantly refers to the healer as catalyst. All of them trained students in shorter or longer courses that were usually followed by a time of apprenticeship in very individualized ways. But their influence reached beyond their personal students, and their artistic integrity won them the acknowledgment and respect of the psychiatrists and psychologists with whom they worked.

When in 1965, mainly on Marian Chace's initiative, dance therapists from throughout the United States got together to found the American Dance Therapy Association, it became apparent that the use of movement and dance as a therapeutic tool was not confined to areas and models these pioneers had established.

Already in the forties and fifties a number of dance educators had extended their work with children in creative dance into specialized areas besides that of the emotionally disturbed, such as the blind, the deaf, and multihandicapped children. An early pioneer in work with deaf children is Elizabeth Polk, an Austrian-trained dancer and educator, who for years worked in institutions with groups and individuals. Hilda Midlin, too, worked with a wide range of children, from the normal to the emotionally disturbed and defective, and based her efforts on a systematic use of child development theory as well as close cooperation with psychologists and psychiatrists. Blanche Evan belongs in this group too. In her private studio, which has served for many years as a dance center for children and adults, she developed dance therapy in close cooperation with doctors and psychiatrists. Here she conducts patient sessions and trains dancers in her approach to dance therapy. She is also affiliated with special dance education in the New York University School of Dance Education.

Another influence on the development of dance or movement therapy came from individual psychiatrists who stress body-mind unity. This led to a number of approaches, among them the use of body movement by the psychiatrist or psychologist himself in conjunction with verbal therapy. Dr. Alexander Lowen, a psychiatrist trained by Wilhelm Reich, developed in years of experimentation, together with a group of coworkers, diagnostic and treatment procedures based on physiological concepts of muscle tension and Reichian concepts of muscle armor. The fusion of body-mind principles in treatment is condensed into the "bioenergetic" method. Lowen has trained psychiatrists as well as movement therapists. His physical methods have aroused both controversy and enthusiastic acceptance among dance therapists. His writings have reached and influenced a great many therapists working with movement. A quote from one of his lectures helps explain his work:

> It is an axiom of bioenergetic analysis that a person can only feel his body. One cannot feel the environment except through its effect upon the body. In reality then, one feels how one's body reacts to the environment or to external objects and perception of this feeling is projected upon the stimulus. . . . All our feelings are body perceptions. How much we feel and how deeply we feel is a function of self-awareness.

This stress on feeling through one's body and the vital importance of the flow of unrestricted breath confirms the insights of many individual dance therapists, though they may have arrived at it by means of the more holistic tool of dance.

In contrast, Dr. Judy Kestenberg sees the role of the dance therapist as complementary to the psychotherapist. Her concern is with observing body movement in children and adults. She has crystallized these observations around the theory of child development by Anna Freud and her group of child analysts. She uses Laban's Effort/Shape theory to trace the development of children from the newborn to school age. The "profile" of movement variations she obtains from these observations parallels the developmental scale of Anna Freud. Her concern with the newborn became extended to the child-mother relationship, the physical interaction of mother and child. She uses the dance or movement therapist to train mothers, maintaining a strict separation between verbal and nonverbal bodily re-education. The common ground between psychiatrist and movement therapist is the vocabulary of Effort/Shape terms, which should enable the psychiatrist to give specific prescription and the movement therapist to work and to discuss the patient within this common vocabulary.

It would far surpass the intent of this article to describe all variations of the body-mind approach used either by psychologist or psychiatrist or by dance therapists. There are a number of dance therapists who work close to psychiatric concepts, and there also are a number of psychotherapists who make use of body movement in conjunction with verbal approaches. Some, like Albert Pesso and Elaine Siegel, use techniques that are close to psychodrama and derive from psychoanalysis of Freudian orientation.

The founding of the ADTA has revealed a spectrum of relationships between dance therapist and psychotherapist. Wherever their work was fruitful together, it seems that it was based on a working out and determination of respective contributions—a situation which is still rare, though it exists, as some of the papers and reports from ADTA conferences indicate. The rapid expansion of the group of dance therapists cannot in itself be taken as an indication of a unified theoretical and clinical state of dance therapy or of its acceptance in the professional world.

However, the variety of approaches and groups that feed into dance therapy; the increasing number of agencies other than mental institutions—rehabilitation centers, daycare centers, prisons, drug-addiction centers, halfway houses, out-patient clinics; the work with different age groups—young children, school children, adolescents, adults, and the elderly, attest to increased needs based on changing concepts in all of therapy and social work.

There is a whole spectrum of attitudes toward nonverbal behavior and dance therapy among psychotherapists, ranging from a completely negative evaluation of its usefulness to neutral acceptance of dance activity, along with other recreational modalities, in a hospital program because of its socializing values to acknowledging dance as a modality in its own terms. The latter view is an outgrowth of close cooperation over a number of years within a therapeutic team. The work of Beth Kalish, Sharon Chaiklin, Janet Adler, and Mildred Hill and others in the East; of Alma Hawkins, Trudi Schoop, Joan Smallwood on the West coast reflects this cooperation. In such work a common ground is established, where concepts like body attitude, body image, self-identity, communication, interaction, ritualization, symbolic representation are shared but have specific meaning within each modality. They are considered or agreed upon as important for both therapeutic approaches in improving functional living.

On the other hand, among the practitioners of movement there exists a wide variety of degree to which they base their therapeutic work on psychiatric, psychoanalytic, or psychological concepts.The interchangeble use of the terms "dance" therapy, "movement" therapy, "psychomotor" therapy reflects the groping orientation toward the vocabulary and concepts of psychotherapy which developed therapeutic interference from a verbal model. Albert Pesso, in Boston, and Elaine Siegel, in the New York area, for instance, emphasize the psychoanalytical base of their work.

To this author—speaking strictly personally as an oldtimer who has watched the scene of dance therapy—it seems essential for the psychotherapist and the movement practitioner both to achieve a deepening understanding of the range of dance as the art of behavior which encompasses more than one level. The "holy" madness of the individual artist and the emphasis on the spectacular aspects of theatrical display constitute merely one side of dance. The other side is composed of the regulatory, interactional forces of the dance that include more than expression of emotion. This second aspect we may call here community dance. It occurs still as an alive force in cultures not dominated by technology—as in many parts of Africa, for instance. It is a central force in the forming and regulating of group and individual relationships, interaction, and definition of role. In Western culture it has been almost extinguished or has faded into a fringe socializing role. Some elements of it seem to emerge at this moment in certain avant-garde dance and theatre. An awareness of it is traceable also in the changing attitudes of mental institutions, toward mental illness, and in social work.

With increasing frequency the point is stated that early childhood and adult deprivation of the arts are, in general, a factor in mental illness and social unrest. There is a recognition of the importance of the deprivation of those stimuli that are the source of creativity in the arts, in inventiveness, and in planning activities of the community. This attitude, this author feels, may well be a decisive factor in the development of dance therapy, in determining if it is to move essentially toward methods of changing specific behavior or whether it will serve in a multifaceted way to lead the individual back to creative functioning in the community. But whether the development goes toward educating and re-educating creative resources or toward specific methodologies adapted to a particular psychopathology, the dance therapist finds himself balanced between the arts and sciences. He, therefore, will need a common vocabulary in which elements of nonverbal aspects of expression and communication can be identified and described. This point was first raised by Harris Chaiklin at the 1968 annual conference of ADTA and aroused a lively debate when Paul Korngetz, a New York psychologist, pleaded for a movement theory in the introductory speech of the 1971 ADTA convention. In the discussion, the issue of whether Effort/Shape was such a theory became an acute matter around which a variety of attitudes toward dance therapy and its philosophy or theory were expressed. One outcome was the title and planning of this year's conference: "What Is Dance Therapy, Really?"

It would surpass the intent of this article to say more about Effort/Shape in relation to dance therapy. One remark, though, is needed to clear a frequent misunderstanding. Those of us in the dance therapy field using Effort/Shape see in it not a method of therapy but a tool of increasing sensitivity to movement responses and direct communication. Its usage has convinced us that we do not yet fully understand the entire range of nonverbal behavior; nor could we claim that Effort/Shape is the panacea in specialized methods of therapy. But a theory of movement that is not merely a borrowing from the verbally oriented psychological and psychiatric vocabulary seems a vital factor in establishing methods and in enabling the therapist to make specific contributions to research, while maintaining his intermediate position between the arts and sciences.

Among the developments that have been considerably accelerated by the forming of the ADTA is the increase in training programs for dance therapists. Particularly in dance departments of universities and colleges, undergraduate or graduate programs in dance therapy are being planned or established. It speaks for the fluidity and vitality of the whole field that the most recent programs show different faces: Wynelle Delaney at Texas Institute for Child Psychiatry (Texas Children's Hospital) has founded a four-year program for community health workers for healthy children and adults; the master in Dance Therapy Program at Hunter College, New York City, under Claire Schmais and Elissa White orients students toward the psychotic patient in therapy, research, and evaluation; and Dr. Alma Hawkins is planning a dance-therapy program that would provide a balance between art and science resources.

The ADTA, under Sharon Chaiklin as its president, has intensified and accelerated the efforts gradually building and solidifying a new profession, which until recently was done only in the isolated and individual work of the pioneer and second-generation dance therapists. The direction it will takc is likely to be far from unified; its vitality, however, promises a variety of training and therapy models, filling a variety of clinical, educational, and community needs. It also provides quite a number of dance therapists who have worked in relative isolation with opportunities for sharing and exchanging professional and administrative problems. Standards of work and professionalism are still at great variance in this vast country. Reading the proceedings since 1967 of the ADTA annual conferences makes one realize that problems and growth in a new field are closely related, hopefully as necessary steps of development.

Dance therapy has received encouragement, warning, challenges, and advice. Professor Hans Falck has written in the *National Associaton of Social Work Newsletter* (Vol. XI, No. 3) that

> Dance therapy is a new professon, and new professions—unlike other institutionalized ones—can still make choices about their future directions, their theoretical logic, their intellectual stance in educating neophytes. It is, therefore, pertinent to ask whether dance therapy ought to develop as a sub-specialty to medicine, thereby committing itself to a disease model approach; or, whether it would flourish and be true to its essential logic by orienting itself to the social sciences, to group work in social work, i.e. to an interactional model? Is it, in other words, really a "therapy" or a social intervention? As we have said, it can make that choice.

Dr. Harris Chaiklin also pointed out at the third annual conference of the ADTA in 1968 that

> Dance therapy can accomplish the wedding of art and science by paying close attention to the standards it adopts. If it wants to be a profession, then it should show it right from the beginning, use a role definition which reflects this. The three role attributes which are the hallmark of a profession are service, teaching, and scholarship.

I am looking forward as I write this to the seventh annual conference of the ADTA, with its theme, "What Is Dance Therapy, Really?," in Santa Monica, California, where, in presentations of approaches and of theory, the profession will try to come to grips with what Harris Chaiklin called in 1968 "the difficult task of finding out what it knows, what it doesn't know, and what it needs to know." This will be the first conference on the West coast. Alma Hawkins, who had been the most active link between the East and West coasts, has been instrumental in the planning of this conference. The vastness of the United States makes it difficult to communicate and to have a comprehensive picture of dance therapy while being moored in one's own area. The author may, therefore, be forgiven if names and descriptions of therapies are incomplete. It is one person's view from one's own horizon of intensive involvement. If she were asked what is the chief difference between dance therapy and teaching dance, her one sentence answer would be: The former has to do with evoking movement response, the latter with being trained in a skill.

In Memoriam—Marian Chace

Long ago, there was a woman.
  A smile through a wreath of smoke
A touch gentle for wounds
  firm for strengths—
A body large yet not large,
  strong yet fluid—
And feet always seeming above
  the ground.
Then there was a girl, not
  yet a woman—
There was silence between them—
The girl was filled with words
  which could not be said,
With darkness.
Woman and girl heard a
  song one day.
Suddenly hand touched hand,
  and music like a lightening bolt
drew from the still figure
  a faltering step—
The woman smiled
  The girl smiled back—
Day after day this silent
  communion was
Until finally to some simple song
Girl, woman and music built
  a dance—
Feet weak; arms leaden,
  tense and bitter still,
As Orpheus led the bride
  back from Hell,
So now for years rather than
  for days
The girl followed these
  loving feet—
Soon there were words, soon
  there was work to do
Then there was a goodbye—
All that was twenty years ago—
  Now the woman is dead—
the girl can dance no more—
But God who took the one
  and fiercely yet gently still
  pursues the other—
Knows what the outcome will be.

Eithne Tabor

PROFESSIONAL BIOGRAPHY OF MARIAN CHACE

Pembroke, 1 year, Liberal Arts
Corcoran School of Art, 1 year
Denishawn School, 5 years
Dalcroze Eurhythmics, under Elsa Findley, New York City 5 years
Martha Graham, 2 years
Wigman School—Hanya Holm and Louise Kloepper, 2 years
Music theory and music history with private teachers during the period as head of own concert group

EDUCATION RELATING TO PROFESSIONAL CAREER AT SAINT ELIZABETHS HOSPITAL:

Basic Psychiatry, Washington School of Psychiatry, and Related Courses under Frieda Fromm-Reichmann, 2 years
Clinical Conferences and Classes at Saint Elizabeths Hospital, from 1942 to the present time
3 Seminars in recreation relating to the arts, Washington School of Psychiatry
Continuing attendance at hospital teaching clinics

PROFESSIONAL EXPERIENCE PRIOR TO SAINT ELIZABETHS:

1 year concert tour with own company
3 years as member of Denishawn Concert Company
2 years teacher of children at Denishawn School of Dance
12 years director of own concert dance school
12 years director of own concert dance group. Various concerts for civic affairs, University of Virginia, other groups, personal concerts, etc.

PROFESSIONAL EXPERIENCE AT SAINT ELIZABETHS AND CHESTNUT LODGE:

20 years dance therapist at Saint Elizabeths Hospital
20 years dance therapist at Chestnut Lodge, Rockville, Md.
Lecturer at various hospitals, clinics, and universities in the United States
Director of dance therapy workshop in New York City 8 years
Volunteer work in dance at Saint Elizabeths Hospital, 1 year

Part-time member of Red Cross Staff, doing dance therapy at Saint Elizabeths Hospital, 1 year

Full-time member of Red Cross Staff, doing dance therapy at Saint Elizabeths Hospital, 3 years

Member of Saint Elizabeths Staff, Psychotherapy Section, as Music Supervisor and Dance Therapist, 20 years

Dance Director at Chestnut Lodge, Rockville, Maryland, 20 years

Member of faculty for the group work training program. Sessions held with the group work trainees in communication in body movement

Lecture demonstrations for various student and staff groups in dance therapy on a continuing basis

Conferences on dance therapy with numerous visitors who are interested in dance as non-verbal communication

Supervision of volunteers who are learning dance therapy as well as assisting

Training of students who are voluntary but will stay for periods of time

Recipient of the outstanding service and the Oveta Culp Hobby awards in 1955

Director and teacher of dance therapy workshop in Israel at the invitation of the Rubin Academy of Music in Jerusalem, the official school of Israel

Lectures to professional people in Jerusalem and Tel Aviv

PATIENT PRODUCTIONS:

Producer and director of creative productions from 1953 to the present time. These productions are presented to audiences of patients, staff and public during Mental Health Week.

Director of television production of "Cry of Humanity."

Director of performances for the chapel at a candlelight service for Christmas from 1958 to the present time

Retired from Saint Elizabeths—October 31, 1966
Died—July 19, 1970

BIBLIOGRAPHY

ARTICLES

Chace, Marian. "Rhythm in Movement as Used in St. Elizabeth's Hospital." *Group Psychotherapy, A Symposium.* Edited by J. L. Moreno. Beacon, New York: Beacon House, Inc., 1945. Pp. 243-245.

——. "Dance Therapy at Saint Elizabeth's Hospital." *The Psychiatric Aide*, 8 (September, 1951), pp. 3-4.

——. "Opening Doors Through Dance." *Journal of the American Association for Health, Physical Education, and Recreation,* 23 (March, 1952), pp. 10-11, 34, 39.

——. "Physiological Aspects." *Music Therapy,* 2 (1952), pp. 63-67.
Presented as "Personal Gratification Through Music Participation." National Association for Music Therapy, Topeka, Kansas, 1952.

——. "Techniques for the Use of Dance as a Group Therapy." *Music Therapy,* 3 (1953), pp. 62-67.
Presented at National Association for Music Therapy Conference. Lansing, Michigan, 1953.

——."Dance as an Adjunctive Therapy With Hospitalized Mental Patients." *Bulletin of the Menninger Clinic,* 17 (November, 1953), pp. 219-225.
Reprinted in *Impulse,* 1 (July, 1954), pp. 14-18.

——. "Dancing Helps Patients Make Initial Contacts." *Mental Hospitals,* 5 (February, 1954), pp. 4-6.

——. "Common Principles in Music Therapy." *Music Therapy,* 4 (1954), pp. 87-90.

——. "Report of Group Project, Saint Elizabeth's Hospital." *Music Therapy,* 4 (1954), pp. 187-190.

——. "Hotel Saint Elizabeth: A Unique Experiment in Therapy." *Americas,* 7 (May, 1955), pp. 33-36.

——. "Dance Therapy for the Mentally Ill." *Dance Magazine,* 6 (June 1956), pp. 37-39, 58.

——. "Measurable and Intangible Aspects of Dance Sessions." *Music Therapy,* 7 (1957), pp. 151-156.
Related to "A Psychological Study as Applied to Dance." Presented at American Psychological Association, New York City, 1957.

——. "Development of Group Interaction Through Dance." *Progress in Psychotherapy–Technique of Psychiatry.* Vol. 3, Edited by J.H. Masserman and J.L. Moreno. New York: Grune and Stratton, Inc., 1958. Pp. 149-153.

——. Stimulation of Creative Forms in Patient Production." *Bulletin of the National Association for Music Therapy,* 7 (September, 1958), pp. 9-10.
Presented at Southeastern Chapter of National Association For Music Therapy, March, 1958.

——. "Dance in Growth or Treatment Settings." *Music Therapy,* 8 (1958). pp. 119-122.
Reprinted in *Conflict in the Classroom.* Edited by Nicholas J. Long, William G. Morse and Ruth G. Newman. Belmont, California: Wadsworth Publishing Co., Inc., 1965. Pp. 209-211.

——. "The Role of the Psychiatric Nurse in Dance Sessions." *SNANYS Newsletter*, 8 (October, 1960), pp. 8-9.

——. "A Note on Dance Therapy." *Group Psychotherapy*, 13 (September-December, 1960), p. 205.

——. "The Contribution of Dance in the Education of Children: The Need for Communication and Creative Release for the Individual." *Quality and Quantity in American Education.* Forty-Sixth Annual Schoolman's Week Proceedings. Edited by Frederick C. Gruber. Philadelphia: University of Pennsylvania Press, 1960. Pp. 221-225.

——. "Leadership in Dance Sessions Within an Institutional Setting." *Yearbook of Brooklyn College Association for Health and Physical Education*, 2, (October, 1961), pp. 20-23, 27-28.

——. and Bunney, Judith R. "Some Observations on the Psychodrama Sessions at Chestnut Lodge." *Eighth Annual Chestnut Lodge Symposium*. Rockville, Maryland, 1962. Pp. 19-31.

——. "The Structuring of Dance Session for Varying Needs of Patients." *Music Therapy*, 12 (1962), pp. 63-68.

——. "The Power of Movement with Others." *Dance Magazine*, 38 (June, 1964), pp. 42-45, 68-69.
Presented at American Psychiatric Association, Los Angeles, 1953, as "Use of Dance Action in A group Setting."

——. "Dance Alone is Not Enough. . ." *Dance Magazine*, 38 (July 1964), pp. 46-47, 58-59.

——. "Music In Dance Therapy." *Music Journal*, 25 (November 1967), pp. 25, 67.

——. "Untitled Article on Professional History." *Journal of the American Dance Therapy Association*, 1 (Fall, 1968), pp. 2-4.

Dyrud, Jarl E. and Chace, Marian. "Movement and Personality." American Dance Therapy Association. *Proceedings of Third Annual Conference*. Madison, Wisconsin, 1968. Pp. 16-20.

Chace, Marian. "Movement Communication with Children." American Dance Therapy Associaton. *Proceedings of Third Annual Conference*. Madison, Wisconsin, 1968. Pp. 60-63. In conjunction with a film of the same title produced by Sandoz Pharmaceutical Laboratories.

PANEL DISCUSSIONS

Chace, Marian, Clark, Vernon, Cohen, George M., and Pathman, Julian. "The Role of the Arts in Therapy." *The Northwestern University Reviewing Stand*, 17 (November 11, 1951), pp. 3-9.

——. and Johnson, Warren R. "Our Real Lives are Lived in Movement." *Journal of Health, Physical Education, and Recreation*, 32 (November, 1961), pp. 30-32, 56. Comments Selected by Bettie Jane Wooten.

Dyrud, Jarl E., Chace, Marian, and Erdman, Jean. "The Meaning of Movement: As Human Expression and As Artistic Communication. American Dance Therapy Association. *Proceedings of Third Annual Conference*. Madison, Wisconsin, 1968. pp. 1-15.

UNPUBLISHED

——. "A Psychological Study as Applied to Dance." American Psychological Association, New York City, 1957. Related to "Measurable and Intangible Aspects of Dance Sessions." *Music Therapy*, 7 (1957), pp. 151-156.

——. The Arts and Mental Illness. Interdisciplinary Conference, Saint Elizabeth's Hospital, 1959.
——. "Dance Therapy for Adults." National Education Association Conference, Division of Dance and Therapeutics, Atlantic City, 1961.
——. "Leadership in Dance Sessions Within the Institutional Setting. District of Columbia Mental Health Association, 1963.
——. "Rhythmic Action for Communication." American Association for Humanistic Psychology, New York, 1966.
——. When Expressive Therapy in the Dance is Contra-Indicated. Lecture-Demonstration. American Association for Humanistic Psychology, New York, 1966.
——. "Talk for Louisiana State Community Ballet Group Conference. March, 1968.
——. "Body Image." Taped April 18, 1970, Houston, Texas.

ABOUT

Ridenour, Norma. "Dancers in the Dark." *The Woman,* 21 (December, 1948), pp. 45-48.
"This Month's Cover." *Mental Hospitals,* 5 (June, 1954), p. 3.
Stern, Edith M. "She Breaks Through Invisible Walls." *Mental Hygiene,* 41 (July 1957), pp. 361-371.
Stern, E.M. "Dance of Release." *Coronet,* 45 (January, 1959), pp. 96-100.
Time, February 23, 1959, pp. 60-62.
"Dancing Back to Reality." *Roche Medical Image,* 1 (Spring, 1959), pp. 5-7.
"Dance Therapy Initiated in Israel." *Music Educators Journal,* 51 (February-March, 1965), p. 130.
DeFreitas, Laura. "In Memoriam. Marian Chase." *American Dance Therapy Association Newsletter,* 4 (September, 1970), pp. 1-2.
Tabor, Eithne. "In Memoriam: Marian Chace." *American Dance Therapy Association Newsletter,* 4 (September, 1970), p. 3.
American Dance Therapy Association. "In Memoriam. Marian Chace, 1896-1970." *Dance Magazine,* 44 (September, 1970), p. 90.
Bennion, Barbara. "Marian Chace Memorial, October 23, 1970". *American Dance Therapy Association Newsletter,* 4 (December, 1970), p. 1.
Bartenieff, Irmgard. "A Post Conference Letter To the American Dance Therapy Association." *American Dance Therapy Association Newsletter* 4 (December,1970), pp. 10-13.
Pasternak, Catherine. "Marian Chace." American Dance Therapy Association. *Proceedings of Fifth Annual Conference.* New York, 1970. Pp. vii-xii.
Dyrud, Jarl E. "Marian Chace." American Dance Therapy Association. *Proceedings of Fifth Annual Conference.* New York, 1970. P. xiii.
Toombs, Mary R. "In Memoriam—Marian Chace." *Journal of Music Therapy,* 7 (Winter, 1970), p. 144.
Bartenieff, Irmgard. "Dance Therapy: A New Profession or a Rediscovery of an Ancient Role of the Dance?" *Dance Scope,* 7 (Fall/Winter, 1972-1973), pp. 6-18.